Working with Global Aphasia

Global aphasia is the most severe and disabling form of aphasia, yet it has had the least attention within aphasia research and rehabilitation. This practical book provides the reader with a comprehensive understanding of the topic based on both clinical observations and the literature to date. Uniquely, it covers not only the severe language impairments observed in global aphasia but also the co-occurring cognitive impairments that often present an additional challenge when working with this population.

This book offers:

- A comprehensive understanding of the clinical characteristics of global aphasia illustrated with real case examples
- A theoretical overview of the domains of cognition and discussion of the role cognitive deficits play in the clinical presentation of people with global aphasia
- Critical analysis of the research evidence on global aphasia
- An exploration into the strengths and limitations of common methods used to assess language, cognition, and functional communication in global aphasia
- New ways of approaching assessment and treatment which consider the impact of cognitive difficulties
- Detailed suggestions of direct and indirect treatment tasks and approaches that can be used with this population, including novel cognitive tasks.

This accessible text will provide both experienced speech and language therapists and students new to the subject with the knowledge, skills, and tools to work effectively with people with global aphasia in a range of clinical settings. It will also be an essential resource for anyone considering research with this challenging but highly rewarding population.

Sharon Adjei-Nicol is a highly experienced speech and language therapist specialising in global aphasia. She worked across a range of settings with adult clients during her 15-year career with the NHS. She now runs an independent speech and language therapy practice, Acquire Speech and Language Therapy, where she works with clients with neurological and voice conditions. She was awarded her PhD in 2020 after completing research in the area of global aphasia and is a part-time senior lecturer in speech and language therapy at the University of Greenwich.

The *Working With* Series

The *Working With* series provides speech and language therapists with a range of 'go-to' resources, full of well-sourced, up-to-date information regarding specific disorders. Underpinned by robust theoretical foundations and supported by intervention options and exercises, every book ensures that the reader has access to the latest thinking regarding diagnosis, management and treatment options.

Written in a fully accessible style, each book bridges theory and practice and offers ready-to-use and well-rehearsed practical material, including guidance on interventions, management advice, and therapeutic resources for the client, parent or carer. The series is an invaluable resource for practitioners, whether speech and language therapy students, or more experienced clinicians.

Books in the series include
Working with Children's Language, 2nd edition
Diana Williams
2022 / pb: 9780367467913

Working with Voice Disorders: Theory and Practice, 3rd edition
Stephanie Martin
2021 / pb: 9780863889462

Working with Communication and Swallowing Difficulties in Older Adults
Rebecca Allwood
2022 / pb: 9780367524784

Working with Solution Focused Brief Therapy in Healthcare Settings
Kidge Burns and Sarah Northcott
2022 / pb: 9780367435097

Working with Children Experiencing Speech and Language Disorders in a Bilingual Context
Sean Pert
2022 / pb: 9780367646301

Working with Global Aphasia
Sharon Adjei-Nicol
2023 / pb: 9781032019437

Working with Global Aphasia

Theory and Practice

Sharon Adjei-Nicol

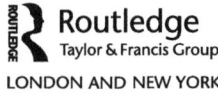
Routledge
Taylor & Francis Group

LONDON AND NEW YORK

Designed cover image: © Getty Images

First published 2023
by Routledge
4 Park Square, Milton Park, Abingdon, Oxon OX14 4RN

and by Routledge
605 Third Avenue, New York, NY 10158

Routledge is an imprint of the Taylor & Francis Group, an informa business

© 2023 Sharon Adjei-Nicol

British Library Cataloguing-in-Publication Data
A catalogue record for this book is available from the British Library

Library of Congress Cataloging-in-Publication Data
A catalog record for this book has been requested

ISBN: 978-1-032-02667-1 (hbk)
ISBN: 978-1-032-01943-7 (pbk)
ISBN: 978-1-003-18452-2 (ebk)

DOI: 10.4324/9781003184522

Typeset in Interstate
by Apex CoVantage, LLC

To Lawrence, Lydia, and Ezra

Contents

Figures

Tables

Preface

Working with my first client with global aphasia was a humbling experience as a newly qualified speech and language therapist. I went along confidently expecting to see improvements. However, I soon realised that this client was very different to others I had seen, so profoundly impaired that I may not be able to effect much change. Indeed, limited gains were made in therapy and neither I nor my colleagues knew what to do. Unfortunately, the evidence base was limited too, with very few books or papers to help. During my years of clinical practice since, many more clients with global aphasia have baffled me, but more importantly, they have challenged and inspired me – first to conduct my PhD research on global aphasia, and then to write this book. Whilst my PhD provided a unique opportunity to gain in-depth knowledge on this subject and try new ways of working with this client group, much of my knowledge has been gained through trial and error with clients and learning from others. I have been fortunate enough to have worked with many outstanding therapists and academics who have influenced and inspired me in different ways. There are too many to name, but some warrant a special mention: my former colleagues at Macclesfield District General Hospital, Barbara Hegarty, Tanya Cavlovic, Joseph Buttell, Suzanne Beeke, and Carol Sacchett.

This book comes nearly 40 years after the only other resource dedicated to this population was produced (*Diagnosis and Treatment of Global Aphasia* by Michael Collins, 1986) and is an attempt to re-explore this complex condition using a modern lens. It is an offering based on everything I have learnt about global aphasia through various people and channels. The content focuses on functional (everyday) communication as well as cognition, an area that has too often been neglected in aphasia. Whilst it does include theory and research findings, the aim is for this book to be a practical clinical resource. Furthermore, the scarcity of evidence and research on global aphasia means that much of what is presented has had to be based on my personal clinical observations and experience. My hope is that this book becomes not only a valuable clinical resource for students and therapists but also a source of motivation for others to consider writing about and conducting research with this challenging but highly rewarding population. There is no doubt that they are in much need of our efforts and expertise.

I will end by thanking my family and friends who have been so patient as I have once again neglected them to focus on writing. Thank you for all your love, support, and encouragement.

Abbreviations

AAC	Augmentative and alternative communication
ABA-2	Apraxia Battery for Adults-2
ASHA-FACS	American Speech and Hearing Association Functional Assessment of Communication Skills
AST	Aphasia Screening Test
BCA	Better Conversations with Aphasia
BCC	Basic choice communicator
BDAE	Boston Diagnostic Aphasia Examination
BNVRT	Butt Non-Verbal Reasoning Test
CADL	Communication Activities of Daily Living
CAT	Comprehensive Aphasia Test
CEBM	Centre for Evidence-Based Medicine
CoBaGa	Cognitive Test Battery for Global Aphasia
CLQT	Cognitive Linguistic Quick Test
COAST	Communication Outcomes After Stroke Scale
COPM	Canadian Occupational Performance Measure
CSC	Controlled situation communicator
GANBA	Global Aphasic Neuropsychological Battery
ICAP	Intensive Comprehensive Aphasia Programme
LARK-2	Language Activity Resource Kit 2
MCA	Middle cerebral artery
MCST-A	Multimodal Communication Screening Task for Persons with Aphasia
MDT	Multidisciplinary team
MIT	Melodic Intonation Therapy
MLE	Milan language examination
MMCT	Multimodal communication training
NMT	Neurologic Music Therapy
NVAFA	Nonverbal visual assessment of flexibility in aphasia

OT	Occupational Therapy
PACE	Promoting Aphasics' Communicative Effectiveness
PICA	Porch Index of Communicative Ability
PPT	Pyramids and Palm Trees Test
PwA	People with aphasia
PwGA	People with global aphasia
PwSA	People with severe aphasia
RCPM	Raven's Coloured Progressive Matrices
RCT	Randomised control trial
SaLT	Speech and language therapist
SA-QOL-39	Stroke and Aphasia Quality of Life Scale-39
SCA	Supported Conversations for Adults with Aphasia
SLT	Speech and language therapy
SPPARC	Supporting Partners of People with Aphasia in Relationships and Conversation
STM	Short term memory
SYCOM	Symbolic Communication Training Through Music
TIDieR	Template for Intervention Description and Replication
VAT	Visual Action Therapy
WAB-R	Western Aphasia Battery-Revised
WCST	Wisconsin Card Sorting Test
WM	Working memory

WHAT IS GLOBAL APHASIA?

Introduction

Aphasia is a condition which refers to an acquired loss or impairment of language function. It can affect comprehension, expression, reading, and writing and is often classified into subtypes based on linguistic features, communication strengths, and communication weaknesses. Goodglass and Kaplan (1972) differentiated between fluent and non-fluent aphasias. They described fluent aphasia as containing frequent uninterrupted periods of speech whereby five or more words might be produced together with relatively spared grammar and articulation. In contrast they described non-fluent aphasia as containing utterances of four words or fewer with a lack of grammatical structures. One type of non-fluent aphasia is global aphasia. Global aphasia is characterised by little to no verbal output (speech) in all conditions (repetition, naming, spontaneous speech) alongside significant auditory comprehension deficits. Of all the aphasia subtypes, global aphasia is the most severe and disabling form. The limited residual language in this type of aphasia can leave clinicians struggling to know where to start in terms of intervention planning and delivery.

To some extent use of the term "global aphasia" has become less favoured in recent years. Frequently "severe aphasia" is used as an umbrella term to include those with global aphasia. However, I use the term severe aphasia to refer to clients who have severe difficulties in one or two communicative domains (such as verbal and written expression) but relatively spared abilities in others (such as comprehension and reading). Global aphasia on the other hand I use to refer to clients who have equally severe deficits across all domains, and it was an intentional decision to name this book "Working with Global Aphasia" rather than "Working with Severe Aphasia." Assessment and treatment approaches can differ greatly between severe and global aphasia and the evidence base is far greater for the former than the latter. This is primarily because people with global aphasia (PwGA) are rarely included

DOI: 10.4324/9781003184522-1

in research studies and have had little attention dedicated to them in the literature. The challenges of assessment, intervention planning, and delivery in a client with both severe receptive *and* expressive difficulties are by far greater than that of a client with some spared skills. To use the same term for both types of client or to consider that intervention for one group can automatically be generalised to another is unhelpful for all. It is perhaps the tendency to presume this that has contributed to the limited resources being available for global aphasia.

There is a need to recognise global aphasia as a distinct condition and design assessment and intervention tools specific to and appropriate for this client group. The last time a book was dedicated to this population was in 1986 when *Diagnosis and Treatment of Global Aphasia* by Michael Collins was published. Since then, research papers, book chapters, and clinical resources relevant to this population have been few and far between. This has left clinicians with little evidence base to use to support their work. It is my hope that this book goes some way towards rectifying this situation.

Global aphasia: a description

Language profile

Generally, in global aphasia, comprehension is limited to understanding a few high frequency nouns or personally relevant vocabulary. However, as with all aphasia subtypes, variability exists and PwGA are not a homogenous group. Boller and Green (1972) assessed comprehension in 15 patients with severe or global aphasia and found that some PwGA were able to distinguish whether a question was delivered in English or a foreign language and whether words were jargon or real. There have also been descriptions of clients who are able to follow one- or two-step bodily commands or understand personally relevant questions and conversations (Goodglass, 1981; Goodglass, Kaplan, & Brand, 1983).

Whilst comprehension abilities amongst those with global aphasia can vary, expressive abilities are consistently poor in all with the condition. It is rare that a picture can be named accurately or a content word/phrase be used in the appropriate context by a person with global aphasia. It is not uncommon to find PwGA have no verbal output whatsoever. Commonly, repetition skills are also limited, but some PwGA can repeat a small number of single words and phrases (Collins, 1986) or produce automatic speech such as counting or reciting the days of the week. Others may produce a few stereotypical utterances by which a phrase might be clearly articulated and have appropriate intonation but be produced without discretion in any or all attempts at speech (regardless of relevance to the context).

For others still, attempts at verbal output may mainly be neologisms/jargon (nonsense words which differ from their target word by more than half of their phonemes). It is important at this point to differentiate between PwGA who produce jargon and those with Wernicke's or jargon aphasia. The distinction mainly constitutes a difference in the amount of verbal output. Whilst a person with global aphasia may produce jargon, they would not be able to do so fluently, that is in streams of more than four words in length. On the other hand, a person with Wernicke's or jargon aphasia may produce phrases and sentences full of jargon and/or other paraphasias.

Even when there is some degree of spoken output in global aphasia, one key issue is the client can rarely use this language consistently or functionally (in real-world, natural contexts). A further issue is that expressive difficulties may be compounded by apraxia of speech which frequently co-occurs with the condition (Goodglass, Kaplan, & Barresi, 2001). Apraxia of speech is characterised as difficulty with coordinating the positioning and sequencing of the muscle movements required for volitional production of speech sounds (Duffy, 2005).

Reading comprehension abilities in global aphasia are usually as impaired as auditory comprehension (Keyserling, Naujokat, Niemann, Huber, & Thron, 1997) and it is rare that use of written words can be used as a strategy to enhance comprehension. Difficulties have been observed in PwGA in tasks such as matching identical letters, matching common written words to pictures, and reading personally relevant single words (Ho, Weiss, Garrett, & Lloyd, 2005; McCall, Shelton, Weinrich, & Cox, 2000; Schuell, Jenkins, & Jimenez-Pabon, 1964).

Global aphasia often occurs with contralateral hemiparesis (weakness and inability to move one side). Frequently, this affects the dominant side for writing and makes this skill even more of a challenge. Some PwGA retain a small amount of residual spelling abilities and can spell personally familiar information such as their name using an alphabet board or their non-dominant hand. However, it is rare that spelling abilities are advanced enough for PwGA to be able to use spelling functionally or through text-based augmentative and alternative communication (AAC). It is not uncommon to see PwGA who have significant difficulty with basic tasks such as copying shapes and letters. Upper limb apraxia (difficulty carrying out purposeful movements with the arms and/or hands) may further reduce ability to use writing and other compensatory methods requiring use of the upper limbs, such as gesture, effectively.

Cognition and functional communication in global aphasia

Historically, people with aphasia (PwA) have been assumed to have intact cognitive and intelligence skills. Cognition has not been a significant part of speech and language therapy (SLT) training or formed a significant part of assessment or treatment focus. In recent years however, more research into and understanding of the link between cognition and successful functional communication has been gained. There is increasing evidence that spared cognitive skills are required for PwA to use compensatory strategies such as writing, gesture, or drawing effectively in real-life situations and to switch between such strategies. McCall et al. (2000) and Morrow-Odom and Swann (2013) describe PwGA who were able to express themselves functionally using gestures and other non-verbal communication skills due to relatively good cognitive skills such as insight, self-awareness, and self-monitoring.

Despite these descriptions, more often than not, clients with global aphasia are unable to use non-verbal communication or compensatory strategies effectively. Even basic functional communication skills such as making a choice can be difficult for many. It is probable that cognitive deficits are playing a part in such difficulties. In Collins' (1986, p. 5) definition of global aphasia, he encapsulates the extent of cognitive deficits that may occur, stating,

> Global aphasia is a severe acquired impairment of communicative ability across all language modalities, and often no single communicative modality is strikingly better than another. Visual nonverbal problem-solving abilities are often severely depressed as well and are usually compatible with language performance.

Despite this definition highlighting the co-occurring cognitive deficits that may be present, few studies have explored this further. Whilst in recent years the importance of cognition for successful functional communication has been recognised in milder aphasias (see for example Ward-Lonergan & Nicholas, 1995; Wallace, Purdy, & Skidmore, 2014; Purdy & Wallace, 2016), there has been relatively little attention into how the cognitive deficits in global aphasia may affect functional communication. Clinical experience suggests that those with global aphasia do not form a homogenous group. There are some who interact socially, communicate basic needs, and contribute to conversation through non-verbal communication and there are others with little to no ability to do this, who are passive and fully reliant on the communication partner to anticipate their needs.

There has been an attempt to distinguish between those PwGA who have relatively spared functional communication and cognitive skills and those who do not. For example, Garrett and Beukelman (cited in Beukelman & Mirenda, 1998, p. 469) described those who have impaired cognitive skills alongside their language difficulties as "Basic-Choice Communicators" (BCCs), that is they have "profound cognitive-linguistic disorders across modalities" and significant difficulties initiating basic communication, responding to conversational input, and responding to non-verbal signals. In other literature terms such as the "aphasic isolate" have been used to describe those presentations on the severe end of the global aphasia spectrum. De Renzi, Colombo, and Scarpa (1991) describe such clients as "bereft of the possibility of entering into any form of communication with other people" and "uninterested in any form of human interchange." A term I have heard used anecdotally to describe this subgroup is "global aphasia plus." Garrett and Beukelman (1998) describe those who may have similarly impaired linguistic skills to BCCs but relatively better cognitive abilities as "controlled situation communicators" (CSCs). CSCs are described as being able to initiate communication acts consistently, participate in routine conversations with familiar others, and indicate needs by spontaneous pointing. Lasker and Garrett (2006) make a distinction based on communication partner dependency. They state some clients can be "partner dependent communicators" who require cueing or assistance to utilise strategies or "independent communicators" who can access and utilise strategies without assistance (p. 218). They describe partner dependent communicators as having "extreme difficulties in speaking, using symbols, and responding to conversational input," as rarely communicating purposefully non-verbally, and as having difficulties recognising objects and photographs. The description of BCCs by Garrett and Beukelman (1998) and partner dependent communicators by Lasker and Garrett (2006) suggests some clients have difficulties beyond the linguistic (language) level in cognitive domains such as visual perception, visual recognition, and non-verbal semantics and that these deficits are leading to difficulties recognising objects and non-verbal signals. The presence and implication of cognitive deficits in global aphasia will be discussed further in Chapter 2.

In summary, global aphasia can be characterised by limited spoken expression in the presence of severely impaired auditory comprehension, written comprehension (reading), and writing (spelling) abilities. There is variation in the residual functional communication abilities of those who fit the definition. A few with global aphasia may have the ability to functionally communicate or use alternative means of communication. However, many cannot and have severe impairments in basic tasks such as object-to-picture matching. This variation is likely due to differences in the degree to which cognition is impaired alongside language in a particular client.

Prevalence and aetiology

Despite being the most severe and disabling form of aphasia, global aphasia has been the least researched of all aphasia subtypes. No information exists on the prevalence of global aphasia. Collins (1986) estimated prevalence to be between 10% and 30% of post stroke aphasia cases. However, this depends on the time at which aphasia is assessed. In the very acute stages many clients present with global aphasia but this may go on to resolve or change into a different form. With medical advances such as the use of thrombolysis in acute stroke, it is possible that prevalence is falling. However, anecdotally chronic global aphasia seems more prevalent in the more elderly stroke patients. With an ageing population nationally and internationally, the condition may continue to be seen regularly clinically and perhaps increase in prevalence.

There have been no recent investigations into the prevalence of global aphasia. Historically, global aphasia has been assumed to occur alongside contralateral hemiparesis after large perisylvian lesions in the territory of the left middle cerebral artery (MCA) affecting both Broca's and Wernicke's area. However, we now know that different patterns of brain damage can induce global aphasia. Ferro (1992) identified five types of damage in a group of 54 PwGA. The most common damage involved either anterior-posterior cortical and subcortical structures or the anterior and superior division of the MCA with lesser damage subcortically. Similarly in a group of 17 PwGA, De Renzi et al. (1991) found that the most frequent presentations inducing global aphasia were an infarct affecting the whole territory of the left MCA (cortical and deep), or damage to the superior branches of the left MCA only. The white matter connections underlying Broca's and Wernicke's regions are slowly being understood to play a more important role in language and specifically speech production than the cortical regions themselves (Dronkers, Plaisant, Iba-Zizen, & Cabanis, 2007; Hope, Seghier, Leff, & Price, 2013). Indeed, both De Renzi et al. (1991) and Ferro (1992) have identified cases of global aphasia where damage is only subcortical with no damage to Wernicke's or Broca's areas. The head of the caudate, putamen, and internal capsule were relevant areas in the De Renzi et al. (1991) study. Global aphasia after lesions affecting only the posterior and parietal branches of the MCA have also been noted but is a less common presentation (De Renzi et al., 1991; Ferro, 1992; Keyserling et al., 1997).

There is some evidence that global aphasia occurs more frequently in women than in men (Hier, Yoon, Mohr, Price, & Wolf, 1994). Of those presenting with acute global aphasia, some will progress to less severe forms within six months to one year (Sarno & Levita, 1981; Ferro, 1992; Mark, Thomas, & Berndt, 1992) whilst in others, global aphasia will persist past one year becoming chronic global aphasia. The exact proportion of people with acute global aphasia who will go on to have chronic global aphasia is unclear. However, some have attempted to predict this based on lesion site. Ferro (1992) in an analysis of the CT scans of 54 PwGA concluded that in those with more extensive damage and subsequently more severe language disturbance, chronic global aphasia was likely to persist. In contrast, those with only anterior or subcortical damage, or global aphasia without hemiparesis, had more favourable outcomes. On the other hand, Mark et al. (1992) in a study of 13 PwGA found no clear relationship between global aphasia recovery and lesion.

Prognosis

The prognosis for recovery from global aphasia has generally been documented to be poor (Schuell et al., 1964; Nagaratnam & McNeil, 1999; Munro & Siyambalapitiya, 2016). However, one must consider what is meant by "recovery." The complete alleviation of symptoms is rare in all forms of aphasia. What perhaps has been the issue is that historically PwGA had not been found to make gains in real-life functional communication. Schuell et al. (1964) described global aphasia as "irreversible aphasic syndrome" and stated that "[t]he characteristics of these patients in treatment is not that they make no gains, but that gains do not become functional" (p. 305). Marshall (1987a, 1987b) suggested that the time and cost of delivering intervention to PwGA was not worthwhile given the limited gains made. He went on to propose that speech and language therapists (SaLTs) should deprioritise this population and instead focus on treating those with milder forms of aphasia. A factor in Marshall (1987b) forming such an opinion was that the treatment studies available at the time all seemed to suggest that the limited gains PwGA may make can be achieved only after substantial doses of intervention. However, much of the focus in intervention studies at the time was on impairment-based intervention. Edelman (1987) rightly argued that the limited gains found in studies of global aphasia at the time may be due to real-life communication not being targeted in therapy and assessment measures being insufficiently sensitive to measure small but significant gains in the population.

When intervention focuses on functional and compensatory-based approaches there have been some positive findings. For example, improvements have been reported in gestural comprehension, auditory comprehension, and functional communication with interventions such as Visual Action Therapy (VAT; Helm-Estabrooks, Fitzpatrick, & Barresi, 1982), remnant picture books (Ho et al., 2005), and non-linguistic cognitive intervention (Adjei-Nicol, 2020) without substantial doses of intervention having to be provided. Despite the promising result of such interventions, these are all small scale studies. In reality it is currently impossible to make an accurate judgement as to whether SLT is effective for PwGA because so few intervention studies include PwGA in the first place or evaluate outcomes using assessments sufficiently sensitive to change in this population. These factors need to be considered in aphasia research going forward.

Case studies

The chapter has highlighted the heterogeneity of PwGA, particularly in terms of functional communication abilities. The final section of this chapter will use three case studies to illustrate the variation in PwGA in more detail.

Table 1.1 Case study 1: Mrs M

Background	
Age 79 She lives in a nursing home. She suffered a left MCA stroke. She previously worked as a music teacher and has a supportive husband who visits daily.	
Informal assessment findings	
Object Naming	0/4 No response
Repetition of words	0/4 No response
Automatic speech (complete counting to 5)	No response
Single word comprehension (match auditory word to object from choice of four)	0/3 No response
Single word comprehension (match auditory word to object from choice of two)	0/3 No response
Match identical objects	0/4 No attempts to pick up or point to items
Yes/no questions (biographical and orientation)	No verbal or non-verbal responses Smiling intermittently

Functional profile

Mrs M makes eye contact and smiles in response to communication attempts from others, but otherwise has little to no communicative intent and sits passively. She has no verbal output and is unable to repeat words or sounds or produce automatic speech such as counting. Vocalisations have been noted only spontaneously when coughing, yawning, or eating. Mrs M does not initiate communication, neither does she use finger pointing, facial expression, or gesture communicatively. She shows signs of limb apraxia. She can use some objects appropriately within context or spontaneously. For example, she will pick up a cup and self-feed something to drink. However, when provided an instruction she shows little to no object recognition or ability to use basic objects.

Mrs M is unable to complete most SLT assessment tasks due to her inability to follow instructions and difficulties initiating pointing. Of note is that Mrs M also has limited joint attention ability and does not share focus (e.g. she does not consistently look in the same direction as the therapist even with maximal prompts) and this is an issue when attempting to assess. On some occasions Mrs M has demonstrated the ability to track a person moving around the room or an object in her line of vision.

Table 1.2 Case study 2: Mr B

Background	
Age 72 He previously worked as a builder. He lives in a nursing home, is estranged from most of his family, and aside from occasional visits from his son, he has very few visitors. He suffered two strokes 18 months apart: left fronto-parietal and left MCA	
Informal assessment findings	
Object Naming	0/10 combination of set phrases and neologisms
Repetition of words	0/10 combination of set phrases and neologisms
Automatic speech with prompt 1, 2, 3 . . . . Automatic speech with prompt Monday, Tuesday	Able to continue 4, 5, 6 before producing neologisms Unable to continue with days of the week and produced set phrase
Yes/no questions (biographical and orientation)	Provides verbal neologistic responses rather than a yes/no. Inconsistent with Yes/No chart.
Single word comprehension (match auditory word to picture from choice of four)	1/5 perseverating on the same picture
Single word comprehension (match auditory word to picture from choice of two)	2/10 perseverative or unrelated errors
Single word comprehension (match auditory word to object from choice of two)	3/10 perseverative or unrelated errors
Match identical objects	5/5
Single word reading (match written word to picture from choice of four)	0/5
Write name	Made strokes on page
Copy shapes	Copied a circle and perseverated on this for further items

Functional profile

Mr B's verbal output is limited to neologisms and occasional set phrases of "that's me" and "funny idea." These set phrases are often produced with the appropriate stress and intonation for the context. Mr B does not show awareness of his speech errors and neither does he appear troubled by the fact he is frequently not understood by others. He always appears in a good mood, smiling and attempting to initiate communication using neologisms, facial expressions, or vague attempts at gestures. Mr B independently uses his wheelchair around the care home and although unable to use iconic gestures functionally is sometimes able to point to objects and use facial expression to communicate needs. For example, he is able to make a choice by pointing between two drinks or two items of clothing (when the actual items are presented). Outside of forced choice functional situations, Mr B shows limited auditory comprehension abilities and relies heavily on context and routine to understand. Previous SLT had trialled gesture and use of a communication chart with Mr B but no progress was made, with severe semantic difficulties and lack of motivation reported to be the primary issues. Mr B was therefore discharged from SLT.

Table 1.3 Case study 3: Mr P

Background	
Age 68 He lives with his wife. He suffered a left MCA stroke. He previously worked as a lawyer and was actively working at the time of his stroke.	
Informal assessment findings	
Object Naming	1/10 no responses, perseverative errors, and occasionally unintelligible attempts

Repetition of words	4/10 groping evident, multiple attempts at words
Automatic speech with prompt 1, 2, 3 . . . . Automatic speech with prompt Monday, Tuesday	Able to continue to 7 without cueing then paraphasias and neologisms noted Able to continue intelligibly to Friday without cueing then perseverating
Yes/no questions (biographical and orientation)	Perseverative verbal responses on "yes" Non-verbal responses inconsistent 4/10
Write name	Illegible attempt
Copy letters	Attempts unrecognisable
Copy shapes	Recognisable attempts made
Formal assessment findings (Aphasia Screening Test; Whurr, 2011)	
Single word comprehension (match auditory word to picture from choice of five)	2/5
Single word comprehension (match auditory word to object from choice of five)	3/5
Written word comprehension (match written word to picture from choice of five)	2/5
Sentence comprehension (match auditory sentence to a picture from choice of five)	0/5
Follow verbal commands	1/5
Functional Profile Mr P has good social skills and often appears to be following conversations, nodding or laughing in the correct places. Mr P has good understanding of his daily routine and can understand calendars and time. He uses a few iconic gestures alongside facial expression, finger pointing, and a pictorial communication chart to express his needs and initiate communication in social situations. However, Mr P struggles to express more complex ideas and can become extremely frustrated. Mr P can follow verbal commands in context and was able to complete some formal assessment. His spontaneous verbal output is limited to single sounds but he can repeat some short, one-syllable words and produce automatic speech. He has characteristics of apraxia of speech.	

All three cases described meet the diagnosis of global aphasia. That is, they all display severe impairments across domains of comprehension, expression, reading, and writing. There appear to be only marginal differences in linguistic abilities between clients on informal assessment, yet the differences in functional communication abilities is significant. Mrs M presents with a profile akin to "global aphasia plus" whereby she appears to have profound issues with non-verbal communication, object recognition, attention, and initiation in addition to language. Mr P on the other hand has some spared non-verbal communication abilities and relatively good semantic skills. He is communicating in many contexts despite his aphasia. Mr B falls somewhere in between in that he attempts non-verbal communication but does not have the semantic skills to do this meaningfully.

Chapter summary

Global aphasia is the most severe form of aphasia and affects all language domains. However, the population does not form a homogenous group. There appears to be significant differences in functional communication abilities and the degree to which semantic and cognitive skills are impaired alongside language in those with the condition. This is evidenced by three case studies described in this chapter. Relatively little attention has been paid to this population in the literature when compared with other forms of aphasia. The consensus from the sparse literature that exists suggests prognosis is poor, but the chapter has highlighted that functional communication improvements after SLT have rarely been investigated and more research with this population is required.

2

COGNITIVE DIFFICULTIES IN GLOBAL APHASIA

Introduction

Chapter 1 highlighted how residual cognitive skills might play a part in determining which PwGA are able to functionally communicate and which are not. The relevance of cognition to successful communication and positive outcome after SLT more generally is becoming more widely understood. This chapter will provide a theoretical overview of cognition and explore in more detail the importance of cognition in communication.

Cognition is known to comprise five elements: attention, perception, memory, executive functions, and language (Helm-Estabrooks, 2002; Cumming, Marshall, & Lazar, 2013). It is now widely accepted that aphasia can co-exist with impairments in any cognitive domain. Kalbe, Reinhold, Brand, Markowitsch, and Kessler (2005) found that 94% of PwA had impairments in at least one cognitive domain in addition to language. There is no clear understanding of how the five cognitive domains interact with each other or whether there is a hierarchical order. However, attention is generally accepted to be the most basic of cognitive domains (Helm-Estabrooks & Holland, 1998; Villard & Kiran, 2017) and executive functioning is considered to be a complex cognitive process, requiring high level functioning (Rende, 2000). It is probable that domains of cognition are interconnected, but no interactive model encompassing all domains of cognition exists and cognitive domains have often been studied separately. This is particularly so in the literature relevant to stroke. Stroke research has primarily focused on the domains of attention and executive function. The reason for this may be that stroke is believed to have a greater negative effect on attention and executive function than other cognitive domains such as memory (Cumming et al., 2013). What we know from neuroimaging studies is that a specific cognitive domain is not localised to one particular brain region but instead involves a network of brain regions.

DOI: 10.4324/9781003184522-2

Three networks relevant to cognitive processing have been identified and described by authors such as Duncan (2010) and Mineroff, Blank, Mahowald, and Fedorenko (2018). The first is the multiple demand network. This is said to involve bilateral prefrontal and parietal cortices and to support executive processes and complex cognitive tasks. Next is a default mode network involving bilateral frontal parietal regions. This is thought to be activated when internally oriented processes occur (such as mind-wandering or reminiscing about the past). The third is a core language network involving left fronto-temporal regions. This is thought to be recruited for linguistic processing (Binder, Desai, Graves, & Conant, 2009; Mattheiss, Levinson, & Graves, 2018; Mineroff et al., 2018). Mineroff et al. (2018) found that complex language tasks may recruit both the language network and the multiple demand network, and Dick et al. (2001) found that syntactic (linguistic) processing involved activations in regions relevant to lexical semantics, memory, attention, and perception. These examples suggest that processing related to a specific cognitive domain is not restricted to one brain region and instead may involve activation in a broad network (including regions associated with a different cognitive process).

This chapter will first provide a brief description of the domains of cognition outside of language, before then exploring clinical practice in global aphasia and how cognition might be assessed and considered when planning intervention.

Cognitive domains

Attention

Attention can be defined as the ability to focus on particular stimuli over time and flexibly manipulate this information (Sohlberg & Mateer, 1987). Attention is arguably the most fundamental of cognitive processes. Helm-Estabrooks (2002) highlighted that a failure to attend results in a failure to process information. A failure to process information can then impact any and all tasks in everyday life. Villard and Kiran (2017) describe how SLT presupposes an ability to maintain basic attention to task stimuli. Often PwGA are assumed to be struggling with tasks or performing poorly due to their language deficits but this is often oversimplifying the issue. The pictures, words, or sentences we provide as stimuli need to be attended to, processed, and encoded before meaning or manipulation can be completed, and It Is possible – and in the context of global aphasia probable – that attention impairments may be limiting the ability of clients to fully process the stimuli in the first place.

The model of attention most referenced in the literature relevant to SLT practice is one proposed by Sohlberg and Mateer (1987). They refer to five subcategories of attention, which are hierarchically ordered in terms of complexity: focused attention, sustained attention, selective attention, alternating attention (also referred to as "switching attention"), and divided attention.

According to the model, focused attention (sometimes described as the ability to orientate attention) is the most basic form of attention. It involves the ability to be drawn to and respond to a particular stimulus. A client who is being presented with a picture but is looking at the SaLT or looking elsewhere in the room might be assumed to have an issue with focused attention.

Sustained attention involves the ability to maintain focus on a stimulus and/or maintain a consistent response during a task. There is no agreed time frame as to what constitutes sustained attention, but it is assumed that one should be able to sustain attention for as long as is required to complete a task (usually a few seconds to many minutes depending on the task).

Selective attention involves the ability to focus or sustain attention on a stimulus while filtering out distractions. This type of attention is fundamental to many SLT tasks. A common requirement is for a client to select a target from an array of options. In order to do so successfully, they must first focus attention on each item in the array and then disregard irrelevant or incorrect options. Clients may wrongly be assumed to have not understood the task or the target word when in fact the issue may be that they have difficulty selectively attending to a target and are distracted by competing targets and items in the array. This is an issue that particularly pertains to being able to use a communication chart effectively.

Alternating attention is the ability to switch focused attention between stimuli. This is required when viewing (scanning) an array of items. In SLT there may be a further demand to view an array, then attend to an auditory instruction and then focus attention back to the array. If the SLT repeats the auditory instruction there may be a need to switch focus again. This type of attention can be demanding for some with global aphasia.

Divided attention is the ability to spontaneously process two types of information. If a client is presented with auditory information whilst simultaneously being presented with visual stimuli this type of attention is required.

PwA have been found to have difficulties with all types of attention. They have been found to perform worse than healthy control participants on tests of focused attention (Robin & Rizzo, 1989), sustained attention (Glosser & Goodglass, 1990; Murray, Holland, & Beeson, 1997), selective attention (Van Mourik, Verschaeve, Boon, Paquier, & van Harskamp, 1992), and divided attention (Glosser & Goodglass, 1990; Erickson, Goldinger, & LaPointe, 1996). Whilst there is no documentation about attention deficits in global aphasia, we can assume that deficits in this area will exist and potentially be more severe than has been described in other populations.

Villard and Kiran (2018) have further found that PwA experience increased fluctuations in their attention compared with healthy control participants and more within-session (moment-to-moment) variability in task performance. In their 2015 study, the same authors found that as complexity of task increased, reaction times of PwA slowed and that some also displayed more between-session (session-to-session) variability as task demand increased. Villard and Kiran (2015) could not find any pattern in the profile of participants who did or did not show increased between-session variability. The authors concluded that the attentional issues and subsequent variability in performance between sessions in PwA has implications for assessment in terms of gaining a representative baseline and for long term outcomes. Only one of their 18 participants in the study had global aphasia and it is therefore impossible to draw conclusions about how the performance of PwGA might change with increased task demands. However, given the severity of impairments it is probable that in this population variability may be exacerbated. Indeed, this is what I have noted clinically. I have found nearly all PwGA to display some degree of moment-to-moment and session-to-session variability. It is important to repeat tasks (even if performed well) within and across sessions to gain a more comprehensive view of variability and how this may impact function.

There is no clear consensus about the cause of the attention deficits in PwA. However, it is understood that we have a finite amount of attention that we can allocate and distribute according to the task demands. It is proposed that PwA are either poor at evaluating how much attention they need to allocate to a task or that they have difficulties distributing their attentional resources appropriately (Tseng, McNeil, & Milenkovic, 1993). Attention allocation difficulties or inefficiencies have been used to explain why some PwA can be variable in their performance or perform better in specific situations. For example, PwA have been found to have better comprehension when speech is presented more slowly than at a normal rate. The argument is that if the issue was their aphasia or purely a linguistic difficulty, then speech being presented at a slower rate would not make a difference to comprehension ability. The fact that this occurred in an experiment by Campbell and McNeil (1985) has been hypothesised to mean that PwA are less able to distribute attention efficiently when information is presented at a normal rate but when they have more time to allocate their attention are better able to do so. Tseng et al. (1993) also found evidence to support this. In PwGA, I have found that slower presentation as well as direct cues (e.g. in the form of moving a client's head or finger pointing where to look) as to where to focus attention can significantly improve performance particularly in formal assessment and allow clients to demonstrate some spared linguistic abilities that would otherwise have gone unnoticed.

Van Mourik et al. (1992) are some of a few researchers who have considered cognition in global aphasia specifically. They state based on clinical experience that PwGA are easily distracted and have reduced attentional capacity and memory. They go on to suggest that it is their impairments in attention and memory that are the critical factor in the client group failing to benefit from SLT interventions. There is anecdotal evidence to support this. For example, when PwGA have received non-linguistic treatments that have indirectly or directly treated attention (see for example Helm-Estabrooks et al., 1982; Adjei-Nicol, 2020), their auditory comprehension has sometimes indirectly improved. The process by which attention training may aid linguistic abilities can be illustrated using an auditory comprehension assessment task as an example. In such a task a client is presented with a word and four pictures and subsequently asked to find the picture that matches the word. The client must first realise that they have to allocate some attention to each picture whilst also allocating some attention to listening to the spoken word presented. If the client has attention deficits, they may have difficulties evaluating the task and/or distributing their attention allocation so that they put all their attention resource to listening to the word or to scanning the pictures. In a task that requires attention to both aspects they then perform poorly. On the other hand, the client may allocate their attention appropriately at this point but have difficulties with the next step, which is selective attention. To perform the task accurately, the client must ignore the distractor (incorrect) pictures that do not match the auditory word and select the target. The client may have difficulties in ignoring the distractors and again perform poorly by selecting incorrect pictures. The SaLT may presume that they failed the task because of poor comprehension of the spoken word. In fact the primary issue is attention, and it is possible that with training in divided, alternating, or selective attention, clients can successfully complete the task and demonstrate that linguistically they could understand the auditory word but the demand on their attention system was hindering their performance. Of course this is not the case for many clients and many perform poorly even when attention is taken into account.

However, it is important for therapists to attempt to ascertain where a breakdown lies and consider attention a potential factor. If attention is deemed a contributory factor, the evidence that treating the domain can improve auditory comprehension is limited but nevertheless promising. Chapter 5 will detail possible intervention tasks for training attention.

Perception

In basic terms, perception is the process of experiencing the environment by recognising and interpreting sensory information. Perception plays a critical role in all day-to-day activities. In SLT both visual and auditory perception may be relied upon.

Visual processing involves the acquisition of visual information through the eyeball, along the optic nerve and the appropriate use of that information. Visual perceptual skills are often required in the therapeutic process in terms of recognising the objects and pictures used as stimuli. As has been discussed earlier, many assessment and therapy tasks in SLT require clients to select an option from an array. This requires perceptual skills in the form of visual searching (Heuer & Hallowell, 2009). Warren (1993) presented a hierarchy of visual processing that demonstrates the complexity of this cognitive domain. Initially, Warren (1993) suggests visual processing skills are dependent on oculomotor control (the ability to move the eyes), visual fields (the area the eye can see at a time), and visual acuity (the sharpness of eyesight). Following this, Warren (1993) suggests that in order to perceive visual stimuli, visual attention is required. Visual attention includes the ability to record all details of a scene in a systematic organised way, as well as pattern recognition – the ability to identify salient features of an object such as colour, shape, texture, and contour. Warren's (1993) hierarchy also demonstrates that higher level skills in the form of visual memory (the ability to visually process information, store it, and recall it later) and visual cognition (the ability to manipulate visual information, integrate it with other sensory information and use contextual cues to obtain meaning from an image) are also required. It is important that clinicians recognise that tasks we may deem as basic such as selecting an object or picture from a word are in fact multifaceted and failure at such task may be due at least in part to skills outside of language. Figure 2.1 provides a visual representation of this hierarchy.

To understand in more detail how objects are recognised, it is helpful to also consider the model of object recognition proposed by Ellis and Young (1996, p. 31). They propose that after an object is presented, there is an *initial representation* stage where the

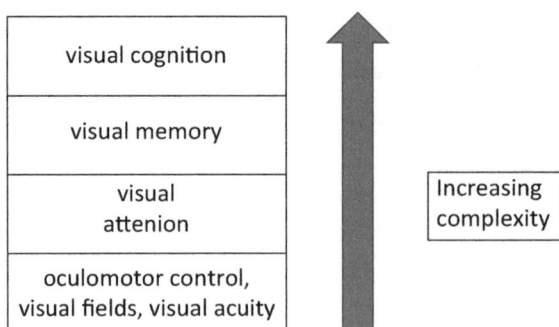

Figure 2.1 A visual representation of Warren's (1993) hierarchical model of visual perception, ascending from low to high complexity

"primal sketch" or two-dimensional geometry of an image is formed. This includes the image's brightness and intensity. Next, *viewer-centred representation* occurs, which involves processing the visible surfaces of the image from the viewer's position. After this there may be a step called *object-centred representation* and then following this *object recognition units* are accessed. Object-centred representation involves the formulation of a three-dimensional representation of the image specifying the shape and surfaces of the object independent of the viewer's position. Object recognition units refers to the stored structural descriptions of known objects. The authors describe object recognition units as acting as an interface between visual and semantic representations. Following access to object recognition units, the semantic system is accessed. This provides information on the object's meaning and allows for the object to be recognised.

Although object recognition issues are noted by the SaLT in clinical settings, often this is interpreted as a semantic issue – a failure to gain meaning from the object. However, it is possible the issue is pre-semantic and more of a visual perceptual issue. For example, the client may have difficulty with recognising two-dimensional forms of objects (as represented on a picture) or difficulty recognising objects when presented at a specific angle. The models by Warren (1993) and Ellis and Young (1996) provide a useful way for clinicians to understand skills underpinning object or picture recognition that can be explored as part of assessment. It is important for clinicians to do this because disorders of perception are common after stroke (Royal College of Physicians (RCP) Intercollegiate Stroke Working Party, 2016) and can impact comprehension and cognitive skills. Problems include missing information in a visual field, slow scanning, difficulty attending to critical features of objects, and agnosia (impaired object recognition) (Humphreys & Riddoch, 1987; Malia & Brannagan, 2014).

There is evidence that in the non-neurologically impaired, language comprehension interacts with visual perceptual processes. For example, studies have shown that when "normal" participants listen to words or sentences that are incongruent with what they are shown visually, reaction time is slower (Kaschak et al., 2005; Meteyard, Bahrami, & Vigliocco, 2007). As has been outlined in the prior section on attention, it is reasonable to assume that in global aphasia the requirement to listen to and comprehend a word/sentence whilst simultaneously visually processing a picture (as in most SLT tasks) may increase cognitive demand to a point where performance on the comprehension task itself may deteriorate.

The literature has paid less attention to auditory perception and auditory attention compared with the visual counterparts of these processes. However, a four stage hierarchical model of auditory perception has been proposed by Goll, Crutch, and Warren (2010). This involves (1) separating what is heard from background noise (auditory scene analysis), (2) encoding the auditory properties such as pitch and timbre (auditory property encoding), (3) processing the acoustic signal and accessing the acoustic representation (auditory object perception), and (4) the recognition of the acoustic data (auditory recognition). Auditory object perception enables auditory data to be processed despite people having different-sounding voices whilst auditory recognition allows us to differentiate among environmental sounds, voice, or music. Goll et al. (2010) suggest that auditory processing can be influenced by top-down processes such as attention, executive functions, and semantics. Auditory agnosia has been described as defective recognition of auditory stimuli (usually environmental sounds) in the context of preserved hearing. Auditory processing difficulties have been reported to be rare, but when they do occur they are usually as a result of stroke and can lead to difficulty perceiving auditory stimuli such as non-verbal environmental sounds and music. (Slevc & Shell, 2015; Simons & Lambon Ralph, 1999). I have encountered PwGA who are unable to differentiate between environmental sounds and speech but this has been very infrequent. The issue was diagnosed only through non-linguistic assessment tasks such as matching an environmental sound to a picture (e.g. match the sound of a drill or the sound of a dog barking to the corresponding picture) and a verification task in which clients are played sound clips and shown a picture that is congruent or incongruent with the clip and asked to verify whether the sound matches the picture by answering "yes" or "no." It is much more common to focus on visual perceptual and semantic tasks within rehabilitation than auditory perceptual and semantics skills, which are largely ignored. Whilst rare, non-linguistic auditory semantic deficits are possible and the model by Goll et al. (2010) provides a useful framework for exploring where a deficit might lie.

Memory

Various models of memory exist and continue to be debated in the literature. For example, the modal model of memory (Atkinson & Shiffrin, 1968) and the Baddeley-Hitch model of memory (Baddeley & Hitch, 1974). It is beyond the scope of this book to discuss them all but through this literature, different types of memory have been discovered. Differentiating between different types of memory is important in clinical practice in order to establish what the demands of a task are and what might be influencing a client's performance. The following section will provide an overview of key classifications within memory.

Memory can be divided into two forms. Verbal memory relates to the ability to remember information presented through words such as names or stories. Visual memory on the other hand relates to the ability to remember things we have seen such as faces, shapes, and maps.

Short term memory (STM) involves storage of information be it visual or auditory, for a brief period of time, usually up to 30 seconds (Baddeley, 2012; Cowan, 2010). If this information needs to be processed or manipulated during the brief period of time it is being stored, then working memory (WM) is required. WM may draw on attention and executive function skills (Murray, Salis, Martin, & Dralle, 2018). Like in attention, STM and WM are considered capacity-limited systems. Memory impairments for both verbal and visual information are common after stroke and can co-occur with aphasia (Snaphaan & de Leeuw, 2007; Bonini & Radanovic, 2015). Brain regions associated with WM include prefrontal and posterior parietal regions (Weintraub et al., 2013) as well as the left superior temporal gyrus (Leff et al., 2009).

In aphasia, STM and WM have been found to be linked to language functions such as sentence comprehension. Leff et al. (2009) found that digit span performance (a test of verbal working memory) predicted performance in spoken sentence comprehension and that the area of the brain relevant for both skills is the left superior temporal gyrus. However, there is no clear evidence of a link between severity of aphasia and severity of memory impairments. Understanding the integrity of memory in severe and global aphasia is extremely difficult because most memory assessments rely heavily on linguistic skills which are of course impaired in this population. WM is however an important skill for functional communication, particularly when language is impaired. Nicholas and Connor (2017) comprehensively discuss the importance of WM for using non-verbal communication or AAC. An example is when using AAC, the client must hold the intended message or need in mind whilst scanning the options available on a chart or within a device.

Long term memory refers to the storage of information for much longer periods of time, that is months, years, decades, or indefinitely. In contrast to short term memory, long term memory does not have a finite capacity. Long term memories can be divided into declarative memory (explicit) and nondeclarative (implicit). Declarative memories require conscious effort to be recalled, whereas nondeclarative memories can be recalled subconsciously. Examples of declarative memories are memories related to events such as birthdays (episodic memories) or those related to general worldly knowledge (semantic memory). Examples of nondeclarative memories are procedural memories (such as how to ride a bike or drive a car) and priming (when exposure to certain stimuli influences the response to stimuli presented later).

Executive functions

Executive functioning is a multidimensional process, consisting of several top-down or supervisory processes that enable goal-directed and adaptive behaviour. However, there is a lack of consensus as to exactly what skills are involved and how they relate to one another (Murray, 2017). Malia and Brannagan (2014) divide executive functions into seven main areas: self-awareness, goal setting, self-initiation, self-inhibition, planning and organising, self-monitoring and self-evaluating, and flexible problem solving (sometimes referred to as "cognitive flexibility").

In recent years executive functioning has received significant attention within the aphasia literature. This is because it is now widely agreed that, second to language, executive functions are the cognitive skills most vulnerable to the effects of brain damage associated with aphasia (Rende, 2000; Helm-Estabrooks, 2002; Cumming et al., 2013). The reason for this is that the blood supply for frontal language structures is shared with the dorsolateral prefrontal cortex, which is an area integral to executive functions (Cumming et al., 2013; Helm-Estabrooks, 2002). Within the domain of executive functions, problem solving and cognitive flexibility have garnered the most interest with respect to aphasia research.

Rende (2000) describes two types of cognitive flexibility. One is reactive flexibility whereby one must freely shift cognition or behaviour in response to changing task or situational demands. The other is spontaneous flexibility, which encompasses the notion of fluency and the ability to produce diverse ideas, consider response alternatives, and modify plans. This is sometimes referred to as "divergent thinking." According to Rende (2000), the two types of flexibility may be differentially impaired. Reactive cognitive flexibility is thought to be particularly relevant to functional communication and the use of compensatory strategies and AAC. This is because using a strategy or AAC in a real-life situation requires the ability to first recognise a problem with getting a message across or with the communication partner interpreting the message and subsequently shifting (switching) to an alternative form of communicating the message. For example, in response to a communication partner not understanding their verbal message or being cued to do so, a client must switch to trying to relay the message through gesture or an AAC device. Miyake and Friedman (2012) suggest that to do this successfully involves the ability to overcome interference or negative priming. In the case of the previous example, because the message that now needs to be conveyed by gesture/AAC would be the same as the one that was previously being attempted via speech, there is likely to be some interference or influence from this. Negative priming is thought to be a cause of perseveration (an unintentional repetition of a previous response). Essentially, perseverative errors are a reflection of an issue with cognitive flexibility. Miyake and Friedman (2012) further propose that to switch successfully, WM must be accessed and any information stored there appropriately revised and updated to accommodate the new requirements of the task. Difficulty updating information in WM may additionally contribute to perseveration.

Given that compensatory communication techniques and AAC are often explored as functional communication options in global aphasia (due to the severity of language impairments), understanding problem-solving and cognitive flexibility skills is beneficial. Unfortunately, despite the high relevance to the population, little to no research has been done on problem solving and cognitive flexibility in global aphasia. In terms of aphasia more broadly, we know that PwA perform worse than non-neurologically impaired controls on measures of visual non-verbal problem solving (Kertesz & McCabe, 1975) - specifically Raven's Coloured Progressive Matrices assessment (RCPM; Raven, 1956) - and worse in terms of speed and efficiency on executive function tests (Purdy, 2002). Purdy (2002) analysed the types of errors PwA made on the Wisconsin Card Sorting Test (WCST; Grant & Berg, 1993), an assessment of executive function, and found they had specific difficulties in initiation of switching behaviour and that they made more perseverative errors. Chiou and Kennedy (2009) investigated cognitive flexibility in 14 PwA (the majority of whom were characterised as having mild aphasia) and healthy controls by varying the conditions in a task which required participants to respond to the command "go" by pressing a button. Sometimes the "go" command would be presented auditorily, other times in writing, and on occasion an extra instruction would be added. These variables could be either predictable or unpredictable. PwA were found to have reduced ability to switch compared with healthy controls. Furthermore, they were slower to switch and made more errors when unpredictable variables were added. Chiou and Kennedy (2009) proposed that such difficulties may negatively affect the ability of PwA to generate different ideas to solve problems, shift from one topic to another, and use a variety of strategies when misunderstood. Whilst the aforementioned studies are not specific to PwGA, we can assume that PwGA would perform similarly to if not worse than the participants in the studies. Consequently, they may struggle even more with the very thing SLT is often aiming to achieve. That is, to switch from relying on speech to get a message across to using other (non-verbal) communication modalities.

The relevance of cognition

The previous section highlights that attention, perception, memory, and executive functions are relevant skills for achieving meaningful gains from intervention and developing functional communication skills. Helm-Estabrooks and Holland (1998, p. 70) stated,

> At the most basic level, therapy requires the ability to attend and concentrate, and memory is critical to all learning. Integrity of visuospatial skills is needed for processing many treatment materials and finally executive skills are required if a patient is to implement and develop ways to communicate in unique situations despite their aphasia.

El Hachioui et al. (2014) demonstrated the importance of cognition to overall functional outcome after stroke. They assessed 147 participants with acute aphasia and found that those with more severe cognitive impairments (difficulties in two or more domains of visual memory, visual semantic association, visual perception, and executive functioning) had a poorer functional outcome as measured by the modified Rankin scale (Bonita & Beaglehole, 1988) than those with milder cognitive impairment (difficulties in fewer than two of the aforementioned domains).

A few studies provide empirical evidence of cognitive deficits in global aphasia. Van Mourik et al. (1992) administered the Global Aphasic Neuropsychological Battery (GANBA), an assessment consisting of five tasks assessing attention, memory, visual and auditory recognition, and intelligence to 17 PwGA. Results suggested the existence of two groups. The first group of four PwGA were found to have intact basic cognitive functions (scoring above 80% on at least four of the GANBA tasks), whilst a larger second group of 13 were found to display variable patterns of deficits including non-verbal auditory processing difficulties, impaired concentration, and a lack of basic visual skills. Van Mourik et al.

(1992) went on to suggest that the first group would be able to benefit from intervention targeting compensatory strategies, such as use of gesture or a communication book. On the other hand, they suggest the second group of 13 who display variable patterns of cognitive deficits may require training in these skills prior to language oriented treatment. They later describe additional unpublished data that suggest a third group exists who appear unmotivated, have little communicative intent and cannot draw, point with intent, or use yes/no consistently. They propose that in this group cognitive and language assessment is impossible and therefore intervention should be indirect and target communication partners and social interaction. In a recent study of six PwGA, Adjei-Nicol (2020) further supports the existence of a subgroup with profound cognitive impairments. At baseline all six participants had difficulties with non-verbal semantics, non-verbal reasoning, selective attention, and executive functioning alongside their aphasia. Furthermore, five of the six participants also made errors at baseline in an object-to-picture matching task, suggesting deficits in basic visual perceptual and recognition skills.

There is evidence of a link between severity of linguistic impairment and severity of cognitive impairments. For example, Kertesz and McCabe (1975) found that participants with more severe comprehension difficulties had more issues with the RCPM (Raven, 1956). Marinelli, Spaccavento, Craca, Marangolo, and Angelelli (2017) investigated 189 PwGA using the Cognitive Test Battery for Global Aphasia (CoBaGa; Maguire, Nicholas, & Zipse, 2012), which is an unpublished non-verbal cognitive battery containing five subtests that evaluate attention, executive functions, logical reasoning, memory, visual-auditory recognition and visuospatial ability. Findings suggested the participants could be divided into three subgroups based on their performance. One subgroup performed well across parameters and had functionally spared cognition, a second group was heterogeneous, demonstrating spared cognitive skills particularly in terms of memory but difficulties in the other areas, and a third group had severe difficulties in all cognitive parameters. Importantly, the authors found that the third group consisted of 39 participants who also had more severe linguistic deficits than the other two groups. Another study with similar findings is that by Olsson, Arvidsson, and Blom Johansson (2019). They divided 47 people with severe aphasia (PwSA) into two groups (verbal and non-verbal) based on their residual abilities and administered subtests from the Cognitive Linguistic Quick Test (CLQT; Helm-Estabrooks, 2001) as well as language and functional communication assessments with each group. They found that the non-verbal group with more impaired verbal language also had more severe executive functioning impairments. As part of a systematic review, Simic, Rochon, Greco, and Martino (2019) examined whether relationships between executive functions and language therapy outcomes were linked to overall aphasia severity. Based on the findings from 15 studies, they concluded that in moderate-severe aphasia, both executive function and language ability at baseline positively correlate with language therapy outcome. That is, executive function skills may be as important as language skills for positive outcomes after SLT in those with more severe aphasias. Van Mourik et al. (1992) have gone a step further and suggested that PwGA with the most severe cognitive deficits cannot benefit from direct SLT at all and should therefore receive only indirect input targeted towards a communication partner and social participation. Whilst the clinical challenge of working with people with severe linguistic and cognitive impairments is a substantial one, the view of Van Mourik et al. (1992) is perhaps overly pessimistic. There is emerging evidence that even those with the most severe forms of global aphasia whom I refer to as having "global aphasia plus" can benefit from SLT, particularly if interventions are non-linguistic and focused on cognitive skills (Adjei-Nicol, 2020). Chapters 4 and 5 discuss intervention in global aphasia and what non-linguistic cognitive approaches might look like. Prior to a SaLT integrating cognitive training into SLT, it is important that they are able to carry out some basic assessments to understand how cognition may be influencing communication. Whilst SLT may wish to work alongside Occupational Therapy (OT) or neuropsychology to establish the exact nature of cognitive impairments (see Chapter 6 for more discussion on joint working), often it is through observation and functional communication assessment that the impact of cognition on communication can be fully understood.

Assessment of cognition in global aphasia

Authors such as Helm-Estabrooks and Albert (2004) and Fridriksson, Nettles, Davis, Morrow, and Montgomery (2006) suggest that SaLTs should spend time assessing cognitive skills in order to improve the quality and success of treatment. Assessment of cognition and in particular executive functioning can be difficult to carry out in people with language impairments and more so PwGA. This section will detail assessments and tasks that I have found useful in clinical practice.

Assessment of attention

Line cancellation tasks are often used to assess attention and visual neglect (Helm-Estabrooks, 2001; Marinelli et al., 2017). They require clients to view a page full of lines that are in different orientations and to cross out with a pen only those that are in a particular orientation. Other permutations of this include a page full of different symbols/pictures with the requirement being to cross out or circle a particular symbol or picture (Helm-Estabrooks, 2001). Some PwGA may find it difficult to follow the instructions and/or use a pen to make a selection. However, others are able to attempt the task, particularly when symbols or pictures are used instead of lines. Analysis of performance will highlight any issues with visual neglect (difficulty orienting or attending to stimuli on one side of the page, usually contralateral to the lesion) and selective attention. In PwGA selective attention difficulties may manifest as the client selecting some or all of the appropriate targets while also selecting distractor/inaccurate stimuli.

The Flanker Task (Eriksen & Eriksen, 1974) is another way of assessing attention in global aphasia. There are various versions of this task, but essentially a target is presented which is flanked by non-target stimuli. The non-targets may be congruent or incongruent with the target. Participants must selectively attend to the target (in the middle position) without being distracted by the flanked items. This test is relatively easy to understand and is non-verbal in nature so has potential for use with PwGA. It has been used in studies with stroke patients and those with aphasia (see for example Kluding, Tseng, & Billinger, 2011; Geranmayeh, Brownsett, & Wise, 2014). Usually the targets are arrows. Figure 2.2 provides a visual example of the task. Online versions of the test exist whereby the client must press the left or right arrow key on a computer keyboard that corresponds with the direction of the target arrow. However, I have often adapted the task to allow clients to make a selection by pointing to a printed copy of a left or right arrow (Adjei-Nicol, 2020). This adaptation can reduce the impact that unfamiliarity with a computer keyboard, visual impairments, or hemiplegia may have. Whilst not all PwGA understand the task, some can complete it. Accuracy has been found to be lower on trials where the "flankers" are incongruent with the target compared with when the flankers are congruent with the target (Ishigami & Klein, 2011) due to difficulties with inhibitory control.

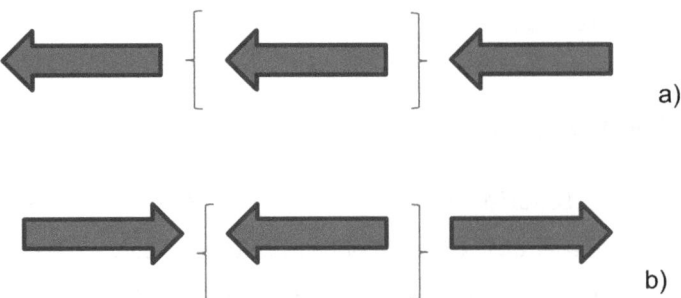

Figure 2.2 A visual example of the Flanker Task: (a) shows the target is congruent with the flanked arrows, and (b) shows the target is incongruent with the flanked arrows

Assessment of visual perception

I have found the initial sections of the Aphasia Screening Test (AST; Whurr, 2011) referred to as "pre-assessment tests" can be a useful screening tool for basic visual perceptual skills. Clients are required to match identical colours, shapes, digits, and letters from a choice of five. There is no requirement to understand the visual stimuli, merely to match them based on their visual properties. If needed, I have reduced the number of items to select from to as few as two. If a client struggles with the task when there are only two items to select from, it is possible that they have severe visual perceptual difficulties. However, it could also be that cognitive impairment is so profound that they do not understand the task requirements. Whilst one can assume that difficulties with basic matching tasks such as those in the AST will mean that perception and recognition of more complex visual stimuli will be more difficult, this is not always the case. In some situations clients find real objects/pictures easier to perceive than shapes, digits, letters, and colours because they may be able to draw on their semantic or conceptual knowledge.

Block design tasks are another way of assessing visual perception in more severe aphasias. First described by Kohs (1920) and later adapted by Wechsler (1955), the task now forms part of many cognitive screening assessments including the cognitive subsection of the Western Aphasia Battery-Revised (WAB-R; Kertesz, 2006). A client is shown a two-dimensional pattern of colours/shapes on a page and required to replicate the pattern with physical (three-dimensional) blocks. I have found that many PwGA find this task difficult. This is possibly because the task does not rely on just visual spatial/visual perceptual skills but also requires an element of problem solving in trying to generate a three-dimensional version of a pattern presented in two dimensions. Limb apraxia may play a further role in some clients struggling. However, the test is standardised and for this reason can be useful to conduct and analyse in specific cases.

Assessment of memory

Digit span tasks are frequently used to assess STM and have been used extensively with PwA (see for example Rönnberg, Larsson, Fogelsjöö, Nilsson, Lindberg, & Ängquist, 1996; Friedmann & Gvion, 2003). Digit forward tasks measure the storage component of memory (STM) by asking clients to repeat digits presented in the same order. Digit backwards tasks require the client to repeat the digits heard in reverse order. This requires manipulation of the material stored and thus relies on WM. In either type of task the client must repeat back strings of increasing longer digits strings and therefore relatively intact spoken output is needed, a skill impossible for most PwGA. However, non-verbal adaptations have been described whereby the participant must point to the correct order of digits on cards rather than verbally produce the order (Friedmann & Gvion, 2003). For PwGA this adapted version may still be challenging as recognition of written digits is required.

In the Comprehensive Aphasia Test (CAT; Swinburn, Porter, & Howard, 2004), there is a memory assessment in which clients are asked to recall pictures previously presented within the assessment from a choice of four, of which three are unrelated distractors. This task can be a useful way of assessing memory without placing demand on linguistic skills.

Assessment of executive functions

The most frequently used assessment of executive functioning in aphasia is the WCST (Grant & Berg, 1948) but tasks such as clock drawing and published assessments such as the Tower of Hanoi (Simon, 1975), Tower of London (Shallice, 1982), and RCPM (Raven, 1956) have all been used to assess this domain.

Clock drawing is commonly used to assess executive function in terms of planning ability (see for example Helm-Estabrooks, 2001) but it also assesses general cognition and visuospatial abilities (Agrell & Dehlin, 1998). It requires the client to draw a clock set at a particular time. The client is then scored based on the presence of specific elements such as symmetrical and accurate placing of numbers. Drawing and semantic memory skills are required to complete this assessment, both of which may be difficult for some PwGA but it is worth a try.

In the WCST (Grant & Berg, 1948) the client is presented with a set of four stimulus cards and asked to sort the remaining (128) response cards without being given further instruction on how to do so. The stimulus cards are similar to the response cards in colour, form, shape, or a combination of these three characteristics. The participants are not told the sorting rules but must determine the correct sorting rule based on feedback. If and when the client correctly sorts ten consecutive cards, the sorting category changes without direct indication from the assessor. The client must recognise the change in feedback and show flexibility of thinking to sort to a new rule. The assessment can be completed without the need for expressive language skills, but the initial instructions can be difficult to follow. This assessment has been used in studies with PwA but many have difficulties with the assessment even when a shorter version of the test (WCST-64; Kongs, Thompson, Iverson, & Heaton, 2000) is used (Fridriksson et al., 2006). I have known only a few PwGA to be able to complete this assessment. However, on the few occasions a client has successfully completed sufficient trials to be able to score the test, detailed information on cognitive skills relevant to SLT can be gained, such as the number of ambiguous versus unambiguous responses, the number of perseverative responses, the number of trials a client takes to understand the task, and more.

RCPM (Raven, 1956) assesses non-verbal visual problem solving by requiring clients to identify the missing element to complete a pattern. The task requirements are relatively simple to explain and can be given non-verbally. No verbal output is required to complete the task. It is possible for some PwGA to complete this assessment as demonstrated by Van Mourik et al. (1992) and Adjei-Nicol (2020) but those on the more severe end of the global aphasia spectrum may struggle. Indeed, Kertesz and McCabe (1975) found a correlation between severity of comprehension deficits and performance on this assessment suggesting those with more severe comprehension deficits will perform worse despite the assessment being non-linguistic. Furthermore, Van Mourik et al. (1992) reported data finding that 31% of PwGA could not complete the RCPM (Raven, 1956) and of those who could, 78% scored at or below the 25th percentile. Generally, I found that PwGA can understand the task requirements but find it challenging so that accuracy is poor.

Keil and Kaszniak (2002) reviewed all available tests of executive function and concluded that the WCST (Grant & Berg, 1948) and RCPM (Raven, 1956) were the most useful for assessing PwA. The authors did not have global aphasia specifically in mind when completing this review and were focused more on whether people with expressive language difficulties would be able to complete the assessments reviewed or not. I would agree that of published and standardised assessments the RCPM is a good option for use with PwGA but the WCST is much more challenging for this group.

The Butt Non-Verbal Reasoning Test (BNVRT; Butt & Bucks, 2004) assesses the ability to problem solve ten photographic scenarios. Importantly, unlike the assessments discussed thus far the stimuli are functionally relevant and real-life scenarios. The client is asked to point to the most appropriate solution from a choice of four photographically presented options. Of the four, one is the target, one semantically connected to the target, one visually connected to the target, and one unrelated. For example, a photo is presented of a woman squinting while holding a letter she is trying to read. The four pictorial solutions to this problem are a pair of glasses (the target), an eye mask (visually related to target), walking stick (semantically related), and a duck (unrelated). Whilst this assessment is useful for understanding executive function skills in the form of reasoning/problem solving, in fact the task relies on more than problem-solving skills. Visual recognition and semantic skills are also required for successful completion of the task. Indeed, the assessment has been found to correlate highly with the Pyramids and Palm Trees Test (PPT; Howard & Patterson, 1992) and to indirectly assess semantic associations as well as problem solving (Butt & Bucks, 2004). Despite its flaws, this is an assessment I use regularly with PwGA due to the simple instructions, task demands, and functional relevance.

Assessment of non-verbal semantics

Given the frequency with which pictures are used as stimuli within SLT, it is necessary to assess whether clients are able to recognise and gain meaning from objects/pictures (something referred to as "central semantics" or "object concepts"). This skill is all too often taken for granted in clinical practice with clients assumed by default to have retained this knowledge. In fact, this is not an uncommon area of impairment in global aphasia. Central semantic issues can mean that when a client performs poorly in any task where objects/pictures are stimuli, poor performance cannot be assumed to be due to comprehension but might be due to failure to understand the picture options presented. Non-verbal visual semantic tests can help clarify whether this is an area of difficulty or not.

Using the PPT (Howard & Patterson, 1992) is an option. A pictorial and written word version of the assessment exists. In the pictorial form, clients are required to match a target picture with another (from a choice of two) based on semantic association. For example, a line drawing of a pair of glasses will be shown as the target picture and a line drawing of an ear as a distractor and an eye as the response. The instructions for this task can be too linguistically complex for PwGA and task demands are high in that the client must look among three pictures (a stimulus/target, target, and distractor), recognise them, understand their meaning, disregard the distractor, and then point to the picture or word best connected with the stimulus. A modified and abridged version of the PPT is contained within the CAT (Swinburn et al., 2004) in which a target picture has to be matched (through semantic association) to one of four pictures. Although the inclusion of four rather than two options puts additional demand on visual processing, in my experience this version is slightly easier for clients to interpret and understand. This is possibly because the inclusion of more pictures provides additional context and enables clients to understand the task requirements more easily. The items used are also in some cases more familiar than in the PPT as are the clarity of pictures. The other positive is that by including a close and distant distractor the therapist is able to make hypotheses about the level of impairment through analysis of errors. Clients' familiarity with items is important to check with family prior to completing semantic assessments. Unfamiliarity through cultural differences may impact performance.

Picture categorisation/sorting tasks can be a simpler way of identifying central semantic deficits, as the instructions are simpler and cognitive demands lower than in the PPT. The client must sort a selection of pictures into piles based on semantic groups. The groups might be distantly semantically related, for example, food versus animals or closely related such as food versus drinks or fruits versus vegetables. An example for each category should be provided and the client asked to place the additional pictures onto the relevant pile. This task is described in Chapter 5 as an intervention task also.

Cognitive screening tools

Screening tests are relatively short assessments that can be useful ways of identifying those with a particular issue and those without. The CLQT (Helm-Estabrooks, 2001) is a screening assessment that tests attention, memory, executive functions, language, and visuospatial skills which can be completed within 15–30 minutes. Whilst the assessment in its entirety will be difficult for most PwGA due to the linguistic demands of tasks such as responding to personal facts, confrontation naming, and paragraph comprehension, some of the non-linguistic tasks such as symbol cancellation, clock drawing, symbol trails, and memory of designs may be possible to complete. The manual of the CLQT allows individual tasks to be scored and analysed separately and therefore useful information on cognitive skills can be gained even when only parts of the assessment are completed.

The following section describes cognitive screening tools that have been described in the literature and used with PwGA but have not been published. Although unavailable to purchase, I have included these as it is possible for clinicians to replicate tasks, and/or follow a similar protocol in clinical practice to gain necessary information about cognition.

Van Mourik et al. (1992) presented the GANBA, which consists of five tasks to assess attention, memory, and intelligence. As the tool was designed for PwGA, there are little to no demands on language in the assessment. It consists of a line cancellation task to assess attention, recognition memory tasks in which objects and faces are the stimuli, a modified version of the RCPM whereby options were presented in a downward column rather than across the page (to ensure clients with neglect or hemianopia can still complete it) as well as matching tasks to assess visual perception. The assessment has been used in a few studies such as Hinckley and Nash (2007) but has not been widely documented. As explained earlier Van Mourik et al. (1992) found that some of their participants could not complete the RCPM (Raven, 1956; Raven, Court, & Raven, 1990) part of the screen and when evaluating the tool the authors suggested it would have been helpful to have included a test of non-verbal semantics such as the PPT (Howard & Patterson, 1992).

Marinelli et al. (2017) and Maguire et al. (2012) have described the Cognitive Test Battery for Global Aphasia (CoBaGa) and the non-verbal visual assessment of flexibility in aphasia (NVAFA) respectively. The CoBaGa is unpublished but made up of five subtests that evaluate attention, executive functions, logical reasoning, memory, visual-auditory recognition and visuospatial ability. It includes widely available assessments such as RCPM (Raven, 1956) as well as letter, digit, and symbol cancellation, a task requiring the client to construct the shape of a human using five cards with different shapes, memory tests using faces and objects as stimuli, as well as visuospatial tasks requiring participants to recognise objects shown in unusual perspectives. Marinelli et al. (2017) describe the assessment tasks in sufficient detail for them to be replicated, and I have particularly found their visuospatial task useful clinically. For example, I will present a mug turned upside down to the client and ask them to match this upside-down object to one of two or three pictures depicting objects in a more familiar orientation. I have encountered PwGA who struggle to complete this task and who can match objects to pictures (i.e. recognise items) only if they are presented in the same direction or from the same perspective as the target. Such a difficulty becomes important to consider functionally and can explain why some clients may struggle to use objects of reference or a picture communication chart.

The NVAFA (Maguire et al., 2012) requires the participant to look at an array of 15 items (either pictured objects or abstract designs). The array is present on ten occasions and each time the items are arranged slightly differently. Every time a page is presented the participant is asked to circle three items that have something in common but must also select three different items to their previous response. As this assessment is unpublished, there is limited information available. I find the instructions complex and have not replicated in clinical practice. However, I have included reference to it in this section because Nicholas and Connor (2017) describe successfully using this assessment with a client with global aphasia.

Face validity in cognitive assessment

The previous section has described ways of assessing different domains of cognition. However, a significant challenge in cognitive assessment is that successful completion of any particular cognitive task often relies on more than one domain. For example, although line cancellation and the Flanker Task purport to assess selective attention, intact visual perceptual skills are also required to complete the task – in the same way a digit span task requiring the client to point to the digits heard relies on intact visual scanning and numerical recognition. I have mentioned already that the BNVRT (Butt & Bucks, 2004) whilst assessing non-verbal reasoning and problems solving is also assessing semantics. To take the WCST (Grant & Berg, 1948) as another example, the client must ascertain the sorting rule (which could be colour, shape, or number) based on feedback they are given after each trial. During the assessment, the sorting rule suddenly changes. Not only is cognitive flexibility necessary, but visual perception skills are also required to sort by colour or shape in the first place, and the participant must be able to switch attention between the task and the examiner to attend to the feedback they have been given. Therefore, when analysing performance in cognitive assessments it is important for the SaLT to consider face validity (the degree to which the assessment measures what it aims to measure) and whether impairments in other cognitive domains may have contributed to poor performance.

Chapter summary

It is difficult to objectively assess aspects of cognition in global aphasia because many tests have complex instructions and task demands or rely on intact cognitive skills such as visual scanning/searching, visual perception, or semantics, which are commonly also impaired in this population. Nevertheless, evidence and clinical experience suggests adapting tasks within the GANBA and CoBaGa and/or completing the following assessments can provide a wealth of information on cognition to support intervention planning in PwGA:

- The Flanker Task (Eriksen & Eriksen, 1974)
- Raven's Coloured Progressive Matrices (RCPM; Raven, 1956–2003)
- Pyramids and Palm Trees Test (Howard & Patterson, 1992)
- Butt Non-Verbal Reasoning Test (Butt & Bucks, 2004)
- Comprehensive Aphasia Test, semantic memory subtest (Swinburn et al., 2004)
- Aphasia Screening Test, Pre-assessment Tests (Whurr, 2011)

3

ASSESSMENT AND INTERVENTION PLANNING

Introduction

Accurate assessment is important for treatment planning and measuring change over time. It is essential that the assessment process allows for both communicative strengths and weaknesses to be captured. Gaining information about communicative strengths is important not just for ascertaining skills that may be able to be utilised in therapy but also for the individual's mood and co-operation through the therapeutic process. PwGA by definition have communication difficulties in all domains and the therapeutic process, particularly in terms of assessment, can be a negative and discouraging one. This chapter will discuss the challenges of assessment in global aphasia and provide suggestions on how to overcome these in order to gain maximal information on language and functional communication skills in this population.

Case history

Prior to any informal or formal assessment, a comprehensive case history should be taken. Ideally, this should be gathered using a combination of information from medical notes and discussion with nurses, doctors, or other multidisciplinary team (MDT) members who have already worked with the client. A direct call or in-person meeting with the client's family or carers can be most beneficial and an opportunity to not only gather information on the client's social history, communication contexts, and pre-morbid communication abilities, but also explain the role of SLT and what to expect from SLT assessment. An attempt should be made to gather information from the client directly using basic yes/no questions and pictures to support comprehension, but in reality this can be difficult with this population, especially in the early stages. The case history stage is vital for understanding the client behind the condition and gaining insight into their linguistic and cultural background,

DOI: 10.4324/9781003184522-3

attitudes, beliefs, and personalities. Wherever possible, the information gained should be used to tailor assessment to the individual client's situations in terms of language preferred for assessment, items and stimuli to be used, and contexts to be observed. For example, if the case history process establishes that a client prayed every day using a particular prayer, the clinician may plan for assessment to include current ability to recite this prayer from memory as in an automatic speech task or read key words within it. Another example may be if the case history establishes that a client spoke to their son weekly on the telephone to advise of what shopping items they required, assessment might include ability to name food items or use a phone. There are some who advocate that goal setting should be completed prior to assessment so that assessment tasks can be tailored to the areas important to the client. I do often use this approach when working with clients with milder aphasias. However, I have found this challenging to do in global aphasia. Often clients with more severe impairments and their families need to be educated about the nature (and severity) of the condition first. Goal setting without understanding of the client's abilities and limitations can be meaningless and daunting. I have found a personalised case history prior to assessment an appropriate middle ground for client-centred assessment in this client group.

Appendix 1 provides suggestions of questions that could be asked within a case history to gain more bespoke information about a client. As mentioned previously, these questions could be asked over the phone or in a face-to-face discussion with a relative or a questionnaire could be left for a relative to complete in written form. Usually, more detail is provided by loved ones when information is sought verbally.

Once information has been obtained from family and other sources, I have found it helpful to ask the client questions from the questionnaire as part of their initial assessment. Sometimes this will demonstrate the severity of the client's impairments, as they are unable to provide any information. Other times clients may be able to verify or refute responses their relative has provided. There is nothing like being told a client likes or dislikes a particular food or television show by a relative and a client vigorously refuting this on checking during assessment. On occasion I will purposely provide information that I know from the case history to be incorrect to see how the client responds. The inclusion of this type of questioning in assessment can be a way to warm up the client to the assessment process and build rapport.

Assessment

Many PwGA retain some insight into their communication difficulties and/or can ascertain through observation of the SaLT's verbal feedback, body language, facial expression, or symbols on score forms (such as ticks and crosses) that they are not performing well. Given the severity of impairments in global aphasia and the likelihood that clients will score at or close to floor in many tasks, the clinician should take care to consider the potential negative emotional impact the assessment process can have on clients and their families. To this end it may be necessary to adapt tasks or instructions so that what little residual skills are present can be demonstrated and some positives found during assessment. Some general considerations to take when assessing PwGA are described by Van Mourik et al. (1992) and further adapted as follows:

- Reduce demands on verbal expression by seeking yes/no responses and accepting non-verbal responses including pointing or manipulation of objects.
- Consider the duration of the assessment session and the client's attention abilities and adapt accordingly. Break up assessment over multiple sessions and/or have breaks between tasks if necessary.
- As discussed in Chapter 2, consider the face validity and the underlying cognitive skills required to complete tasks when interpreting findings. SaLTs should not automatically assume poor performance is due to the client's language impairments.

One of the aims of assessment is to determine skills that can be built on and further enhanced in therapy. This can be determined only if there are tasks that a client *can* perform if not completely accurately, then to some degree during the assessment process. If all assessment tasks are impossible for a client and they perform at floor across the board, then no information is yielded about communicative strengths and the therapist is left with no place to start in planning intervention. I have found the most common issue SaLTs contact me for guidance and support on is knowing where to start when assessment establishes that a client is severely impaired in all areas. In these situations, I encourage the therapist to consider whether any assessment tasks could be broken down and simplified still further. Often, we bind ourselves to the assessment form, just because the form stops at a choice of two. However, what for example happens if there is no choice and a client is asked to "point to the comb" and "comb" is the only picture in front of them? What happens if you demonstrate by saying "comb" then touching the picture before asking them to do the same? Can the client copy you? What happens if you support any potential issues with initiation by gently lifting and guiding the client's hand towards the options? Providing these additional supports can help to establish the cues and support that may need to be integrated into intervention tasks.

When performance in assessment is poor, it is important to first consider the task demands and ascertain what is primarily driving poor performance. It is easy to presume it is the severity of the client's aphasia. However, the cognitive skills required to participate in a typical SLT assessment cannot be underestimated and the clinician must decide whether the issue is purely the client's language impairment or whether the cognitive demands of the assessment task are also contributing.

Just as discussed in Chapter 2 on cognitive assessments, there is an inherent issue with face validity when we think about language assessments. To take a comprehension task as an example, a client must listen to an auditorily presented word and find the picture from a choice of four or five that corresponds to it. This relies on an array of skills beyond just the ability to understand a spoken word. Heuer and Hallowell (2007, 2009) are amongst those who suggest that incorrect responses may be due to the influence of stimulus-driven aspects, such as colour, size, or familiarity of the depicted concepts. They also draw attention to the non-linguistic skills required to complete assessments, namely visual memory, visual attention, object recognition, semantics, and visual search (scanning) skills. Assessment tasks are often purported to assess one language domain but associated non-linguistic cognitive impairments can influence a client's abilities, and alternative explanations for failure or errors are possible.

In global aphasia given the likelihood that cognition is also significantly impacted, the contribution of cognition to performance should always be examined and appropriate assessments completed. If cognition is found to be a factor, then rehabilitation of the relevant cognitive skill can often be as important as the rehabilitation of language skills. This is because in global aphasia (perhaps more so than for other aphasia subtypes), we expect clients to utilise pictures/objects and switch to non-verbal forms of communication. The ability to do this functionally relies heavily on cognition as detailed in the previous chapter. Assessment of cognition has been described in Chapter 2, and this chapter will focus on assessment of language and functional communication.

Assessment of auditory comprehension

The most frequent way auditory comprehension is assessed in global aphasia is by asking a client to listen to a word and then select (usually by pointing) an object or picture that corresponds with it from an array of four or five. Commonly used assessment batteries such as the Western Aphasia Battery-Revised (WAB-R; Kertesz, 2006), Boston Diagnostic Aphasia Examination (BDAE; Goodglass et al., 2001), Aphasia Diagnostic Profiles (Helm-Estabrooks, 1992), Aphasia Screening Test (AST; Whurr, 2011) and Comprehensive Aphasia Test (CAT; Swinburn et al., 2004) all do this. The array may include semantic, phonological, visual, or unrelated distractors. If the PwGA performs poorly, it is usually assumed that auditory comprehension at the single word level is impaired. However, analysis of error types should then be conducted to establish the nature of the impairment and level of breakdown. In clients with milder forms of aphasia it is often easier to see a pattern of performance, for example clients make semantic errors more frequently or benefit from a certain type of cue. More challenging is the common presentation in global aphasia in which a client consistently provides no response or errors are evenly spread among semantic, phonological, and unrelated distractors in an almost random way. In such cases it is easy to assume performance is an indication of the severity of single word comprehension impairments or difficulty understanding the task instructions. However, in my experience a purely linguistic deficit (in the absence of severe cognitive difficulties) rarely leads to no response in a comprehension task. The client with spared cognition can usually draw on pre-morbid worldly/conceptual knowledge, reasoning, and problem-solving abilities to infer the task requirements and provide a guess. However, those with some degree of cognitive impairment may have insufficiently spared semantic or conceptual knowledge to draw on. They may also demonstrate difficulties initiating a response, which is a form of executive function impairment. This may manifest as no responses or the client mimicking the SaLT's demonstration or cues and selecting every picture rather than just one target.

In summary, assessment of comprehension is most commonly carried out through auditory word to picture matching tasks. In global aphasia it is important when analysing performance to consider the nature of errors and *how* the client attempts and performs the task.

Yes/no questions

The client can be asked a variety of questions that require a "yes" or "no" response. Non-verbal yes/no responses in the form of head nodding/shaking or pointing to a Yes/No chart should be accepted. An accurate yes/no response would suggest comprehension of the question. However, as there are only two options of responses (yes or no) chance can play a significant part. To verify responses, the client can be given distractor questions in which the target provided is incorrect. Using a variety of distractors can help pinpoint more specific difficulties. The following example uses a scenario of a client in a hospital setting:

SaLT: Are you in school?
Client: Nods to indicate "yes" (incorrect)
SaLT: Are you in a car?
Client: Shakes head to indicate "no" (correct)

In the previous example, when given an incorrect option (school) that is semantically related to the target (hospital) in that it is also a building, location, and an institution, the client responds incorrectly. However, when given an option more distantly related (car) they respond correctly. This provides the SaLT with the information that there may be some degree of comprehension, but semantics may be an issue. The hypothesis can be further verified with additional examples using a variety of distractors.

Assessing comprehension through yes/no questions can reduce the cognitive demands that might be present when using an array of pictures as stimuli. It allows language to be assessed more crudely but a pre-requisite is ability to provide a yes/no response which in itself is a source of difficulty for many PwGA. When I do use this method, I find it helpful to ask the same yes/no question (i.e. with the same distractor) multiple times to assess for consistency of response and mitigate for chance playing a role in overall score.

Perseverative responses are common in PwGA and in yes/no assessments it can be difficult to differentiate whether an answer is incorrect or perseverative. Another issue is that "yes" and "no" are semantically related concepts. There is subsequently high susceptibility to confusion between the concepts and the reversal or repetition of questions to assess consistency as suggested previously may actually exacerbate this and lead to negative priming and perseveration as discussed in Chapter 2.

One way I have found to reduce the frequency of perseverative responses is to change the order of questions in an assessment. Rather than ask multiple yes/no questions consecutively and then move on to a block of questions assessing another area, I might jump between tasks, asking a yes/no question followed by giving a one-stage command followed by making a request to repeat a word or name a picture. By the end of the assessment, the same number of items would have been presented as in a usual assessment but with the order changed. The other benefit of doing this is that it mimics the attention switching that is required in real-life communication. It is rare that we would ask someone the same type of question multiple times and it is helpful to see how clients respond to the attentional demands of switching between different questions or tasks.

Following whole body commands and commands using objects

The AST (Whurr, 2011) contains a useful subsection of simple commands such as "point to your nose" and "pick up the pen." However, clinicians can also develop their own instructions using objects found in the immediate vicinity as part of an informal assessment. Changing the vocabulary used for commands can be useful, as I find some clients perform differently depending on terminology used. For example, there may be a differential response to commands using the instruction "point to" versus "show me" versus "where is" or "find the." Increasing the length or complexity of instructions can also help ascertain the exact level of breakdown. However, SaLTs should be aware of the limitations of this type of comprehension task. Assessment of the ability to follow multiple stage commands does not provide information wholly relevant to day-to-day functional communication, especially in adults. The frequency of an adult being given an instruction to follow in everyday contexts is low and therefore comprehension of questions, statements, and functional words should always form part of assessment in addition to or in place of command following.

Sentence level comprehension

Sentence comprehension if attempted at all in global aphasia is usually assessed in a similar way to single words. That is, with an auditorily presented sentence and a requirement to find the picture from an array of four or five that best matches the target. Most PwGA would be expected to perform at floor on such a task due to the severity of their language impairments and the length/complexity of the target sentence.

An additional consideration is that to convey sentences, pictures used in sentence comprehension tasks are often complex. The picture must depict actions, multiple objects, and/or people. Consequently, more advanced perceptual skills than those described in the preceding section for single objects are required. It is important to recognise that poor performance on an auditory sentence-to-picture matching task in global aphasia may be explained or exacerbated by visual perceptual difficulties and the inability to correctly perceive or scan multiple complex pictures.

One helpful way to establish if there are underlying cognitive issues is to reduce the task demands by showing only one picture at a time and asking a series of yes/no questions pertaining to the agents, actions, and objects within it.

To take an example from the CAT (Swinburn et al., 2004) as an illustration, one of the target sentences is "The carpet the cat is on is red." The target picture shows a white cat sitting on a red mat. There are three distractor pictures. In the case of wanting to assess sentence comprehension in a client with global aphasia, they could be shown *only* the target picture and asked to answer a series of simpler instructions and/or answer yes/no questions about the picture. For example:

- "Show me the cat."
- "Show me the mat."

- "Is there a cat?"
- "Is the mat red?"
- "Is the cat sitting down?"

Obviously, such adaptations to a formal assessment render the scoring and analysis within the manual ineffectual and the therapist will be able to make only informal anecdotal observations. Nevertheless, given that PwGA would have likely scored at floor on original versions of the task, these modifications at least allow some information to be yielded. Simpler pictures such as verb colour cards could also be used for this task as could a personalised photograph. Caution in the interpretation of yes/no responses should again be exercised because as discussed earlier, there is an element of chance inherent in having just two options as answers. Repetition of the same targets or reversal of questions to assess for consistency can again help. I have found the early sections of the Test for Reception of Grammar-2 (Bishop, 2003) a useful formal assessment to assess sentence comprehension in this population due to the clarity of the photos and simpler grammar and vocabulary used. Some PwGA can complete the early blocks in the assessment whereby two elements, negatives, or basic prepositions "in" and "on" are assessed. As the grammatical construction of the target sentences increase in complexity, PwGA may struggle, and this would be where the modifications outlined earlier such as focusing on one picture within the array may be helpful.

Often SaLTs do not proceed to assessing sentence or paragraph level comprehension in global aphasia because the client has performed poorly at single word level, and it is assumed that this will preclude the client managing sentences. However, not only are sentences more consistent with how the client would have been used to processing language pre-morbidly, but it is also possible that the additional semantic and contextual information provided when a sentence is presented may enhance comprehension. It is very much worth assessing sentence and paragraph level comprehension in this population. An additional factor is that when personally relevant information is used within assessment tasks, receptive performance has been found to improve (Goodglass, 1981; Goodglass et al., 1983; Wapner & Gardner, 1979). Whilst we can argue that use of personal information, context and conceptual knowledge to aid comprehension compromises the integrity of a language assessment, there is also the argument that doing so supports the clinician in intervention planning by establishing the client's residual skills and strategies that aid their performance.

The CAT (Swinburn et al., 2004) contains two short stories and assesses comprehension with yes/no questions related to the stories. For PwGA these passages may be too long and complex. However, clinicians can try short statements relevant to the client's context (e.g. stories using familiar names or situations based on communication history questionnaire or discussion with family) and ask yes/no questions related to this. Non-verbal yes/no responses should of course be accepted.

For example:

> **Instruction:** Listen to what I say. Then answer my question with "yes" or "no."
> Example Target: **Anita came to visit after church. She didn't stay long.**
> Example Question #1: Did Sarah visit?
> Example Question #2: Did Anita come here?
> Example Question #3: Did Anita go to the bank?
> Example Question #4: Did Anita stay all day?

One issue that can arise with this type of task is that as more questions are presented in succession, the longer the interval from presentation of the target to response and the more the client has to rely on memory. To circumvent this and ensure as much as possible that comprehension is being assessed the target can be repeated prior to asking each question. So in the previous example, the target "Anita came to visit after church. She didn't stay long." is provided followed by the first question, then the target is provided again before asking the second question and each subsequent question. Even with this adaptation there is an increased demand on WM compared with single words and it may be that this influences performance more than comprehension of the words per se. Ensuring aspects of cognition are assessed alongside language as detailed in the previous chapter will help in establishing if there is a pattern of performance suggestive of a cognitive overlay.

With careful selection of distractors/foils within this task, semantics can also be informally assessed. For example, if a close semantic foil is provided the client may make an error but with more distant foil they do not. Should yes/no responses be challenging for the client, an alternative task is to use a picture scene such as the picture description stimulus from the CAT (Swinburn et al., 2004), the BDAE cookie theft picture (Goodglass et al., 2001), or a personal photo from the client's own selection and ask questions related to the photograph that the client can point to. For example, in a photograph of a family wedding with the bride and groom cutting the cake, the questions might be "Where is there something we eat in the picture?" "Who is the bride?" and "Where is something we use for cutting?" This can help ascertain understanding of functional vocabulary and concepts. Careful consideration of the foils used may also help establish yes/no consistency or semantic abilities.

Assessment of spoken expression

This will inevitably be a challenging area for PwGA. The traditional tasks of naming and spoken word repetition will likely be extremely difficult but are still worth attempting during the assessment process. In an attempt to offer tasks that the client may show some success in, automatic speech such as counting, saying the alphabet, or reciting the days of the week in unison with the SaLT or independently can be tried. In addition, asking the client to complete phrases that may be familiar to them (see Appendix 2) can be a way to elicit single word responses through some automaticity. The client's cultural background and individual preferences should be carefully considered when selecting phrases to use in such a task. What may seem obvious or automatic to one person may not be for another and familiar British sayings may not be well known in other cultures. It is good practice to check with relatives first. Differentiating between the client's performance in naming compared with automatic tasks can be a way of identifying whether apraxia of speech may also be present, as is asking clients to repeat single sounds or produce mouth shapes for a sound. It is worth considering whether specific assessment of apraxia is required using a tool such as Apraxia Battery for Adults-2 (ABA-2; Dabul, 2000). However, it is probable that the client's overall deficits will make this difficult, as task instructions are relatively complex in this assessment.

Assessment of written expression

Commonly used tasks within formal assessments for this domain are written naming or writing to dictation. These are challenging for most PwGA. However, simpler tasks such as completing missing letters within high frequency words and asking clients to write highly familiar words such as their own name or address may highlight some residual writing ability and/or spelling knowledge. The use of texting on a phone, typing on a tablet/ keyboard, or pointing at letters on an alphabet board can be trialled in place of pen/paper to ascertain spelling ability where writing itself is not possible, e.g. due to hemiparesis.

Copying of written words, asking clients to write/type individual letters (graphemes) from dictation or copy individual graphemes are additional ways of assessing basic abilities to recognise or reproduce graphemes.

Assessment of reading

In most language batteries, reading comprehension is assessed by asking clients to match written words or sentences to pictures.

Similar issues to those discussed earlier with respect to auditory comprehension assessment using pictorial stimuli apply. Underlying cognitive skills required to perceive and attend to pictures should be taken into consideration.

In global aphasia it can be useful to assess if clients can recognise words without necessarily understanding them. This can be ascertained by asking clients to find an auditorily presented word from a list of three or four words. Incorporating personally relevant words such as their own name or family names can further draw out residual reading skills that may otherwise be missed. This task might then be followed up by asking the client to match the written word to family photos or finding family names within a list (with no auditory priming).

When clients particularly struggle with reading, it can be beneficial to screen for pre-linguistic skills such as matching identical letters, matching identical written words, or matching identical written sentences. These can all be found in the pre-assessment tests in the AST (Whurr, 2011).

Assessment of non-linguistic expression

Gesture

Given that the aim of intervention with PwGA is often for clients to utilise some form of non-verbal communication, gaining an understanding of non-linguistic expressive skills such as gesture and drawing is helpful during assessment. As discussed in Chapter 1, limb apraxia is a difficulty carrying out purposeful movements with the arms and/or hands. It commonly co-occurs with global aphasia and can manifest as difficulty copying gestures, difficulty producing meaningful gestures on command, or difficulty using objects appropriately (Dovern, Fink, & Weiss, 2012; Hogrefe, Ziegler, Weidinger, & Goldenberg, 2012). Limb apraxia coupled with hemiparesis of the dominant upper limb can mean gesture is extremely difficult for many PwGA. However, assessing this area gives the clinician an idea of the feasibility of using gesture in therapy in the future. The City Gesture Checklist (Caute, Roper, Dipper, & Pritchard, 2017) is a freely available framework for assessing gestural use. It is intended to be used by clinicians when observing a video recording or conversation of a client in a functional communication context. At the end of the assessment a tally of the number of gestures can be completed and the type of gesture (such as pointing versus iconic gesture) most frequently used calculated. I have used this tool with people on the higher end of the global aphasia spectrum effectively. In more severe clients rather than assessing through observation in conversation, I have conducted a task where the client has to gesture the use of an object or picture presented to them and then used the framework to analyse the client's gestural attempts. Taking the time to analyse gestural attempts can help guide if and how gesture might be used in therapy. Gesture assessment is another area where specific care should be taken to ensure cultural differences in iconic gestures are understood.

The CAT (Swinburn et al., 2004) contains a short subtest of gestural use. The client is shown a picture of an item such as a mug or a toothbrush and asked to demonstrate how the item is used. A client with global aphasia may require a physical object and/or additional instructions to be able to complete this task. Comprehension of gesture is not something that is assessed in any of the commonly used assessment batteries. In global aphasia it is a useful addition for SaLTs to include in the informal assessment process. For example, a choice of three or four pictures/objects can be laid out and the SaLT produce an iconic gesture relevant to one of these items. The client is asked to select which picture or object the gesture relates to. Another option, depending on the client's auditory comprehension and yes/no reliability, is a gesture verification task. The SaLT produces a gesture and asks the client yes/no questions verbally or using pictures for cues. For example, after demonstrating the action for drinking, the clinician could either say "Was I drinking?" or show a picture of a cup and ask if the gesture produced matches the picture. Incorrect/foil questions should be embedded into such a task to make it valid.

For successful performance in a gesture comprehension task, semantic knowledge (in terms of object use) is required. Poor performance within this task is therefore an indicator of underlying semantic impairments. Assessment of non-verbal semantics and other aspects of cognition relevant to communication have been described in Chapter 2.

Drawing

Again, this is not an area commonly assessed. However, I have found it useful to include in informal assessment if total communication is likely to be considered as an intervention approach. Communicative drawing requires skills such as conceptualisation of an idea, semantic knowledge, and adequate graphomotor skills (Helm-Estabrooks, Albert, & Nicholas, 2014). Any or all of these may be impaired in global aphasia. The ability to copy shapes, line drawings, or pictures is a helpful informal task but in actual functional contexts, the client will first need to create a mental image of the item (which will likely be in a three-dimensional format) and then transpose this three-dimensional mental image into a two-dimensional drawing. With this in mind, a helpful way to assess the skills relevant to functional drawing is to present an object and then remove it and ask the client to draw a representation of it from their mental image/memory. Analysis of how recognisable the drawing is and the features omitted will provide a baseline for future intervention.

Additional considerations

Throughout the assessment process particularly if using informal approaches, if a client fails a task, step downs should be considered. This will provide the clinician with the most comprehensive picture as to where a client's breakdown might lie. For example, the client may not be able to point to a picture from a spoken word from a choice of four but is able to do so when only two choices are present. Observation as to whether the client is seen visually scanning the page is also helpful.

Altering the nature of the stimuli can also provide additional information. For example, comparing performance when stimuli are presented as a line drawing versus a colour photograph versus a real object can provide useful information as to the most beneficial therapy resources to use. Many clients derive meaning from real objects better than they can from a picture.

A further consideration to bear in mind is that PwGA often have difficulties initiating responses by pointing either due to limb apraxia, cognitive issues, or a combination of both and this may significantly impact performance. Physical hand-over-hand assistance whereby the client's arm is guided towards the page/array of items or the client's hand/fingers shaped by the therapist into a pointing response may be required. Once these supports are provided, some clients are able to provide an accurate response and demonstrate their linguistic abilities.

A final consideration are the assessment items themselves. In a busy clinical setting, it can be quick and easy to use a generic set of picture cards and objects or generic pictures within an app. However, where possible, use of the client's own items (or photos of these) should be trialled. Personalised examples can be the difference between an accurate and inaccurate response being given. This is likely due to personal items enhancing semantic representations.

Assessment of functional communication and quality of life

Existing measures

The aim of a functional assessment is to understand how effectively PwA communicate in real-life, everyday contexts. The aim of quality of life measures on the other hand is to explore how speech and language difficulties affect social and family life. Many commonly used functional and quality of life assessments are too complex to use with PwGA. This is either due to the linguistic demands or types of scenarios assessed. Commonly used functional communication assessments in the UK include the Communicative Abilities in Daily Living (CADL; Holland, 1980, CADL-2; Holland, Frattali, & Fromm, 1999, CADL-3; Holland, Fromm, & Wozniak, 2018) and more recently The Scenario Test: Validated in the UK (Hilari & Dipper, 2020). Both of these tools rely on the client engaging in role-play with the SaLT and require the ability to understand relatively complex information or questions and then apply them to an abstract (unrelated to the here and now) situation. This will be a challenge for most PwGA. A further issue with assessments that use role play is that they do not measure actual real-life communicative performance. Instead, the client's potential in real life is inferred from their performance in the simulated role-play scenario. It is important to be aware that even if a client with global aphasia can complete such assessments, performance in a simulated scenario may not equate to real-life communicative abilities. It may be that the additional context and semantic information from a real-life setting as well as an actual necessity/intent to communicate leads to a more effective communication. On the other hand, the attentional demands required in real-life contexts (such as the need to ignore background noise and irrelevant visual stimuli or speak to an unfamiliar person) may negatively impact performance when compared with abilities in a role-play setting. Therefore, wherever possible, functional communication should be assessed through both role-play/simulated situations and observation in natural environments.

Other commonly used functional communication and quality of life assessments require performance or confidence in a range of real-life tasks to be rated by the person with aphasia. Examples include the Communication Disability Profile (Swinburn, Byng, & Firenza, 2006), The Living with Aphasia: Framework for Outcome Measurement (Kagan et al., 2008), Stroke and Aphasia Quality of Life Scale-39 (SA-QOL-39; Hilari, Byng, Lamping, & Smith, 2003) and Communication Outcomes After Stroke Scale (COAST; Long, Hesketh, & Bowen, 2009). However, even when aphasia friendly formats that include symbols, pictures, simplified language, and large boldfaced font are used, these questionnaires remain inaccessible for PwGA and they are unable to complete them themselves. It is possible a significant other could do this on their behalf, but when we are considering how one feels about their aphasia, the validity and appropriateness of a proxy completing ratings is questionable.

A further problematic issue with many existing functional and quality of life measures is that the communication situations explored are too advanced to be relevant to the daily life of someone with severe communication deficits. This was an issue raised many decades ago by Houghton, Towey, & Pettit (1982) and remains relevant today. Situations assessed or rated might be whether the client can follow a newspaper headline, participate in a group conversation, or talk on the phone. These are all beyond the capabilities of most PwGA. One assessment that does consider basic communication relevant to PwGA is the Multimodal Communication Screening Task for Persons with Aphasia (MCST-A; Garrett & Lasker, 2005). The tool was designed to determine candidacy for AAC in global aphasia and assesses ability to relay messages such as hunger, tiredness, or wanting a light turned on using symbols or pictures. These are more relevant functional situations for many PwGA and a reason why despite the assessment not having been psychometrically tested or intended for use in this way, I frequently adapt it and use it as a functional communication measure for this population.

The lack of inclusion of basic communication behaviours within functional communication assessments is problematic for use in global aphasia. Of existing formal/standardised functional communication measures, I have found the American Speech and Hearing Association Functional Assessment of Communication Skills (ASHA-FACS; Frattali, Thompson, Holland, Wohl, & Ferketic, 1995) to be the most useful for assessing functional communication skills relevant to PwGA. The assessment asks a significant other to assess the amount of assistance/prompting a client requires to carry out 43 behaviours that include basic skills such as recognising familiar faces, understanding facial expressions, understanding tone of voice, answering yes/no questions, and making wants and needs known. In addition, the ASHA-FACS (Frattali et al., 1995) measures qualitative communication parameters such as the promptness and appropriateness of communication and how much of a burden the communication partner carries in interactions. These are highly relevant factors to consider in people with more severe aphasias and useful as a baseline measure. Despite the positives of this assessment, it is an indirect measure requiring a proxy to rate performance.

Informal assessment of basic functional communication

To my knowledge there are no published tools that directly measure basic functional communication abilities that might be relevant to PwGA (such as responding to a social greeting, making a choice in a functional situation, giving an accurate yes/no response, or sharing joint focus). This is therefore something I do informally through natural observation or through engaging in a basic activity with the client (such as looking through a newspaper or family photo album or playing a game such as Connect 4 or Snap).

In these activities I assess the client's ability to make a choice of task, answer yes/no questions, initiate communication, and understand the rules of a game. I also informally assess functional problem solving through questions and purposeful errors/problems. For example, after the client selects which activity they would like to do, I might then offer them the incorrect option that they did not choose and observe if and how they respond to this. I might "accidentally" place the newspaper upside down and ascertain if the client recognises this and attempts to turn it round. I might call "Snap" to suggest two cards match in a snap card game when they do not, or I might refer to a relative in a photo album by the wrong name and observe the client's reaction.

As there is an element of problem solving inherent to many aspects of communication (such as recognising one is thirsty and that one must therefore request something to drink) it is helpful to include assessment of functional problem solving within communication assessment. This can be assessed through natural observation but there is no guarantee that a problem will arise during the time the SaLT is observing, and the client's communicative potential might therefore missed. By putting in place situations (albeit somewhat unrealistic) the client's communicative potential can be ascertained. When analysing performance in such activities, it is helpful in global aphasia to measure the speed of response and level of prompting or cueing required alongside accuracy. A scale such as in Table 3.1 could be used at baseline and again at the end of intervention as an outcome measure.

Comparing a client's performance in the same scenario using the same stimuli and distractors/problems before and after SLT intervention is a useful functional outcome measure. Often this will demonstrate subtle improvements or changes that might not otherwise be captured in language assessments or rating scales. It is important to take careful note of what stimuli, distractors, prompts, and problems were provided in the assessment so that these can be replicated.

An example of a 5-point rating scale for assessing functional communication is provided in Table 3.1.

Observation of the client in a session with members of the MDT can further enhance understanding of their functional communication abilities. Physiotherapy and OT sessions are particularly useful to observe, and it is not uncommon to find clients initiating more frequently or responding more accurately in situations in which physical stimuli is being used such as touch or, as in the case of OT, there is more context in the form of real objects.

In summary, thus far this chapter has highlighted that whilst formal assessment may be helpful and necessary for diagnosing global aphasia, in order to draw out information on

Table 3.1 An example rating scale for measuring functional communication in global aphasia

Scenario and stimuli used

Behaviour or response to be elicited	Does so without prompting 5	Does so with minimal prompts 4	Does so with significant prompts 3	Response is ambiguous or difficult to interpret 2	Response is inaccurate 1	Does not demonstrate behaviour/ respond despite all prompts 0
Makes eye contact with SaLT Provides a non-verbal Yes/No response						

residual skills, informal assessment is necessary. The chapter has provided examples of relevant tasks for inclusion in informal language and functional communication assessments in this population. Combining these with cognitive assessment tasks presented in Chapter 2 should enable clinicians to have a comprehensive understanding of a client's residual abilities, the core issues driving their difficulties (language, cognition, or both) and how these impairments may impact the client in functional communication contexts. The following section will describe how assessment findings can be used to plan SLT intervention.

Intervention planning

The intervention planning stage requires the synthesis of case history and assessment findings into an understanding of a client's linguistic and functional communication strengths and weaknesses. This information should then be used to support the provision of personalised education to clients and their families. Many might suggest that goal setting should be the next step in the intervention process; however, I have found that in order to ensure that a client or their relatives can make informed decisions about rehabilitation goals and priorities they need an understanding of the condition and SLT process.

Education

Some PwGA will have insight into their difficulties and an ability to understand basic education about the condition if this information is tailored to their communication level. For others, the education may have to be provided to relatives. Whilst generic information leaflets or websites are a helpful start for providing relatives with an overview, I believe global aphasia to require special individualised explanation. The severity and breadth of impairments may not be captured in generic information about aphasia. This may lead to relatives having inaccurate or unrealistic beliefs about their loved one's abilities, their trying to implement strategies suggested on the leaflets that are not helpful for their loved one, or both. Wherever possible, in-person education should be provided using a combination of leaflets, websites, and personalised examples from the client's own assessment. It is important to gauge through responses of the client and their relatives their understanding and acceptance of information and to consider the amount and level of detail to provide. For some, a leaflet may be too overwhelming, and for others, not specific or detailed enough. For some, the inclusion of client specific assessment findings may be helpful, and for others, very upsetting. In the acute stages the shock of the situation may limit the ability of relatives and clients to take on board information and it may be that information is given in small doses and expanded on over time. Education about global aphasia should be provided in a balanced way and care taken to include positive findings from assessment and hope for improvement. It is important to have assessed basic language and cognitive and functional skills in order to be able to find some positive residual skills to draw on in this discussion. If only standardised tools have been used or a generic informal assessment aimed at a client with moderate aphasia it may be difficult to find any strengths or areas of ability.

Care should also be taken to consider the beliefs and cultural background of the client and family in delivering information. In many cases, prior to providing any education I ask the relative what they understand by stroke, what they believe to be the client's main area of difficulty, and what they think recovery/rehabilitation will look like. Sometimes this may highlight religious or cultural beliefs about stroke or rehabilitation that I must be sensitive to in the delivery of education.

The question always asked in client and family education sessions is that of prognosis. As with all aphasias this is difficult to provide. It is true that the evidence suggests prognosis is poor in global aphasia but as touched on in Chapter 1 and will be discussed again in Chapter 4, the evidence in global aphasia is based on only a handful of studies. More often than not, PwGA are excluded from research studies and very few aphasia interventions or approaches have been designed with this population in mind. I always try to explain this fact to relatives. When dealing with people in the acute and sub-acute phases it is important to keep an open mind about the degree to which speech/language may improve. It is possible for global aphasia to transform into other milder aphasia subtypes or to resolve quite quickly in the early stages. Once it becomes more chronic (arbitrarily the consensus seems to be the six-month point), significant improvement is less likely, but gradual small changes in language and communication skills are possible over many years.

A further consideration when providing education is to tailor the explanation to discuss the difference between speech versus language versus communication. The sparse existing evidence suggests that improvement in verbal speech/language skills in chronic global aphasia is low. However, prognosis for comprehension and communication more broadly is on the whole more positive. Obviously, this is not always what families want to hear and reliance on non-verbal communication is never one's preference, but the need to balance hope with realism is important and explaining the benefit of non-verbal communication is necessary. It can be helpful to frame discussion about prognosis and use of non-verbal communication or AAC using other clients as examples to further provide hope. Providing written information or links to sources for clients/relatives to refer to is extremely helpful. I am always surprised at how often relatives are provided with only verbal information by SaLTs. Given the overwhelming situation many relatives are in, not all information delivered verbally may be fully absorbed or remembered and ideally websites or resources for further reading should be provided. I also find that providing a selection of websites rather than allowing relatives to search the internet themselves can help to ensure information they read is appropriate and relevant to their loved one's case.

Goal setting

Goal setting is a way of identifying and agreeing the priorities and expected outcomes of intervention. The National Clinical Guideline for Stroke (Royal College of Physicians Intercollegiate Stroke Working Party [RCP], 2016) advises that goal setting should involve the person with stroke and their family/carers where appropriate, and be measured and evaluated in a consistent and standardised way.

Involving clients with global aphasia in the goal setting process can be difficult for obvious reasons related to their cognitive and communicative impairments and this is acknowledged within the RCP (2016) guideline. However, it is always important to attempt to involve clients where possible.

Talking Mats can be an extremely useful resource for this. It provides a simple 3-point visual scale using picture symbols to reflect a scale of difficulty, importance, or preference. Examples of the 3-point scale include "Difficult/OK/Easy" and "Important/I Don't Know/ Not Important." The client is then provided with various symbols or pictures (one at a time) that represent items related to the concept being discussed. When used for goal setting, pictures representing communication activities (such as writing, using a laptop, and speaking on the phone) can be presented one at a time and the scale related to importance used. The client is asked to place each picture option under the symbol that best reflects their opinion on that item. For example, they may place the picture representing writing under the symbol for "Not Important," the picture representing speaking on the phone under the symbol for "I Don't Know," and the picture representing using an iPad under the symbol for "Important." This would indicate using an iPad as a goal for therapy.

The Talking Mats resources contain a wealth of small symbol cards that can be used for a wide variety of topics as well as symbols to represent the 3-point scale. In some cases, personalised pictures/symbols may need to be created. However, the SaLT will know this only if time is taken prior to the goal setting discussion to consider the most appropriate options the particular client will require. Liaising with family and reviewing the information on the communication history questionnaire (see Appendix 1) can help with selecting items that will be relevant to the client. Using the Talking Mats framework for goal setting does not involve a significant demand on language for the client. The use of a simplified 3-point visual scale rather than numerical scale with multiple levels reduces the demand on cognition as does the process of presenting and focusing on one option at a time. I have successfully used Talking Mats for goal setting and decision making with many PwGA and studies have also shown that people with little or no speech can use the resource (Murphy, 1998a; Murphy, 1998b, Murphy & Boa, 2012). As an outcome measure the tool can be useful for demonstrating changes in client self-ratings. For example, "using my iPad" might be placed under the symbol for "Difficult" at baseline but at the end of intervention be placed under the symbol for "Easy," demonstrating improvement from the client's perspective.

Using Talking Mats alongside the Canadian Occupational Performance Measure (COPM; Law et al., 2019) is a highly effective way to support the development of goals in global aphasia. The COPM is intended to be used as an outcome measure and usually requires a therapist to interview a client and gather information about what they want to do, need to do, or are expected to do in daily life. To garner this information in PwGA, I use the communication history questionnaire (see Appendix 1) and particularly the question asking for a breakdown of a typical day in the client's life alongside liaising with family and use of Talking Mats. The next step in the process of the COPM is to ask the client whether they are able to do each activity and how satisfied they feel with their performance in the particular activity. Again, Talking Mats can be used for this stage. However, the concept of satisfaction may be difficult for clients to understand so I often use a scale related to difficulty instead. The next step of the COPM is for the client to rate the importance of each activity on a 10-point scale but again this can be adapted using Talking Mats and a simpler scale. The next steps within the COPM require the client to select the five most important activities or areas, score their current ability to perform the task, and provide a rating of their satisfaction with their current performance. This stage is impossible for most PwGA and requires significant adaptation such as a visual scale (see Appendix 3) but is possible with some. Usually I take each activity (picture) that the client has placed under the symbol for "Difficult" in turn and ask the client Yes/No questions as to whether they would like to work on this in SLT or not. Those that the client answers "Yes" to become the focus of SLT intervention. Of course, there are some clients where this process is not possible and goals must be set by the SaLT in conjunction with family. Where goal setting with the client is completed, jointly completing these steps with OT can be extremely beneficial, as often activities selected by clients are multifaceted and require an MDT approach. For example, if a goal is for a client to attend a social group, then aside from communication goals related to how the client will understand and interact whilst there, OT and physiotherapy can help support physical aspects such as the client getting there and being able to use facilities such as the bathroom as well as cognitive aspects such as attention and memory.

The acronym SMART has been used in rehabilitation to conceptualise goals to be specific, measurable, achievable, relevant or realistic, and time bound. Due to the need to meet the components of SMART, goals can at times be long, impersonal, or overly focused on changes that can be quantified numerically. More recent discussion in the literature promotes a more relaxed approach to wording (Dorfler & Kulnik, 2020) and being creative in how goals are evaluated. Hersch, Worrall, Howe, Sherratt, & Davidson (2012) promote a SMARTER approach to goal setting which is shared, monitored, accessible, relevant, transparent, evolving, and relationship-centred and focused on collaboration and the holistic nature of people's goals. One important concept within the SMARTER framework is that of evolving goals. Often in clinical practice goals are set for a specific time frame and reviewed at the end but it is more beneficial to review goals in every session or intermittently within a block of treatment to reflect the changing nature of the client's priorities, abilities, and perspectives as they come to terms with their aphasia and understand the therapeutic process more.

A survey conducted with UK-based SaLTs who work with PwGA (Adjei, 2015) identified that the most common goals set were for clients to be able to do the following:

- Express their basic needs
- Indicate "yes" or "no" reliably in response to a question about wants, needs, or feelings
- Make a choice in a functional context such as during washing, dressing, or during mealtimes

Example goals

The following section takes the case studies described in Chapter 1 and details how the comments and priorities of relatives/carers were developed into goals for SLT.

Case study 1: Mrs M

Husband's comment during goal discussion: "I just want her to be able to engage with me. I don't think she even knows I am there most of the time."

- Goal 1: For Mrs M to engage in looking at a family photo album with her husband for ten minutes, showing signs of joint focus and understanding of the activity by turning pages and scanning photos
- Goal 2: For Mrs M to be able to use a Yes/No chart to respond to basic verification questions within structured activities
- Goal 3: For Mrs M to be able to engage in a picture sorting task with her husband on three occasions, showing signs of turn taking and correctly sorting at least half of the pictures by category

Case study 2: Mr B

Comments from Mr B's carer and son during goal discussion: "I never really know what he is saying or what he wants," and "I would love to be able to understand him, if he could just make himself understood."

- Goal 1: For Mr B to be able to express feelings (happy, sad, bored, tired) and ten basic needs (including drink, toilet, go out, bed) using a communication book containing two pictorial options per page
- Goal 2: For Mr B to be able to use a Yes/No chart to respond to questions about his day in supported conversations
- Goal 3: For Mr B to be able to recognise and produce five gestures relevant to his daily routine and needs within appropriate contexts

Case study 3: Mr P

Mr P was able to engage in goal setting with the use of Talking Mats and the COPM. He identified "speaking to his wife and daughter," "reading," "writing," and "using his iPad" as important to him.

- Goal 1: For Mr P to be able to understand written key words and phrases in his personalised communication book

- Goal 2: For Mr P to be able to use total communication to engage in conversations with his wife
- Goal 3: For Mr P to be able to verbally produce targeted single words and set phrases in appropriate contexts

When setting goals, it is helpful to be specific about the exact items, words, or phrases that will be targeted. These should of course be relevant to the client and their context. Where possible, target items should be identified with family and carers. For example, for Mr B (Case Study 2) the specific feelings and some of the needs to be targeted are mentioned. It is important to consider the variability within and between sessions in PwGA and it is rare that I would state that a behaviour must be demonstrated consistently/100% of the time. Depending on the severity of the client I may aim for more than half of the time, 75% of the time, or 90% of the time. Often the behaviour within a goal may take many months/blocks of treatment to become consistently accurate. However, gradual improvements could be captured through incremental goal setting enabling the client to experience success.

Breaking down goals

The next step after goal setting is to consider *how* the goal will be targeted. This requires the SaLT to break down the goal into smaller steps and then identify the skills required to complete each step. The client's ability to complete each step must be measured and any problematic skills incorporated into the intervention plan. To take Goal 1 from Case Study 2 (Mr B) as an example:

To express a basic need by selecting from two pictures requires the ability to do the following:

- Move one's gaze across the page from one picture to the next
- Take meaning from the picture (e.g. identify the use of the object)
- Match one picture to the target issue/need they have
- Selectively attend to this target picture and disregard the irrelevant picture
- Use eye or finger pointing to make a selection

The skills underpinning this goal therefore include the following:

- Visual scanning and gaze shifting
- Non-verbal (picture) semantics
- Selective attention
- Problem solving
- Initiation

Thus, the intervention must include practice of all these elements.

Intervention planning also requires the SaLT to have identified any relative strengths from assessment that might be able to be used in therapy. In the case of Mr B, information from Case Study 2 in Chapter 1 indicates some strengths are that he can initiate pointing responses in assessment tasks and sometimes uses pointing functionally. He has some semantic skills, as he occasionally points to objects functionally. He also appears to have some basic problem-solving abilities in that he can express his needs at times and finds his way round independently. SLT can attempt to advance these skills further.

The frequency and duration of sessions as well as the time frame for reviewing progress should be considered at the outset. The timing of intervention is an important factor to reflect on. There are many cases in which an SaLT might feel direct intervention is not appropriate and that the client requires more time to come to terms with the situation, and/ or improve medically. In these cases, indirect intervention such as providing strategies or training to their loved one might be considered. However, it is important to note they too may also be struggling emotionally and be unable to take on this responsibility.

National guidelines such as the RCP Intercollegiate Stroke Working Party (2016) suggest clients should be offered 45 minutes of intervention daily if they are able to tolerate this. Given the spectrum of abilities within global aphasia, some clients will be able to tolerate this, whilst others may manage only ten- to 15-minute sessions, especially in the initial stages. A further issue in considering ability to participate are levels of alertness and medical status. It is important to remember that the size and severity of stroke or brain injury that induces global aphasia means a greater likelihood of comorbidities that may limit ability to participate. Low mood may further compromise tolerance as might the client having multiple therapies on the same day such as is often the case on an acute ward.

In designing the intervention and planning specific intervention tasks, the SaLT also needs to explore the available evidence base and consider the most appropriate approaches and tasks for their specific client. The following chapter provides an overview of the evidence base in global aphasia.

Chapter summary

Assessment in global aphasia can be challenging because the majority of existing tools are too complex to provide information on clients' residual skills and insufficiently sensitive to small changes in global aphasia. The chapter has highlighted a few assessments that can be useful for global aphasia (e.g. the AST, Whurr, 2011 and ASHA-FACS, Frattali et al., 1995) and has suggested ways that informal assessment can be carried out to overcome the aforementioned issues. Goal setting has been discussed in detail with clinical examples of goals provided and useful resources to support the process such as Talking Mats and the COPM (Law et al., 2019) suggested.

INTERVENTION IN GLOBAL APHASIA: THE EVIDENCE BASE

Introduction

As healthcare professionals, we are encouraged to use evidence-based practice when planning treatment. Evidence-based practice in healthcare can be defined as "the integration of best research evidence with clinical expertise and patient values" (De Brun, 2013). In the context of global aphasia, there is very little research evidence and clients have severe communication difficulties that limit their ability to provide their perspective and priorities. Consequently, the evidence base in global aphasia is based heavily on clinical experience and consensus. This chapter will summarise the limited intervention research on global aphasia and outline some findings of a UK survey on clinical practice.

Evaluating research evidence

In determining what the "best research evidence" is, clinicians must evaluate both the content and quality of research studies. The Centre for Evidence-Based Medicine (CEBM, 2009) provides a framework for determining the quality of evidence. This is based on a five level hierarchical grading system that is in turn based on study methodology.

Randomised control trials (RCTs) involve participants being randomly allocated to a group and each group then receiving different variations of the independent variable (SLT). So for example, one group might receive SLT approach 1, another group no SLT, and yet another group SLT approach 2. The performance of the different groups is then compared. This is also known as between-subjects design. RCTs are generally agreed to be high quality (Level 1) evidence. Systematic reviews evaluating all the RCTs on a particular topic are considered the highest quality (Level 1a) evidence.

DOI: 10.4324/9781003184522-4

According to the CEBM (2009), Level 2 evidence includes cohort studies (where a group of people are observed over a period of many years and compared with two or more other groups), systematic reviews of cohort studies, and low quality RCTs. The CEBM describes case control studies as Level 3 evidence. These are generally retrospective studies comparing a group of people with and without a condition. A common approach in therapeutic studies is to use a within-subject design whereby rather than compare different groups, one group of participants receive all treatment conditions (e.g. treatment 1, treatment 2, and no treatment) and the group's performance before and after each condition is compared. This too is considered Level 3 evidence. Another approach commonly used in intervention studies is case series. This is considered Level 4 evidence and involves more than one participant being offered a specific treatment and their performance being compared before treatment and after treatment. The key factor in a case series is that analysis and reporting is carried out for each individual separately rather than as a group. Finally, Level 5 evidence is deemed to be expert opinion or case studies.

Critical appraisal tools and templates such as the Template for Intervention Description and Replication (TIDieR; Hoffman, 2014) can provide a structure with which to appraise the reliability, importance, and clinical application of evidence. The TIDieR template specifically focuses on whether studies have provided sufficient information for clinicians to replicate the intervention in clinical practice.

When the evidence base in global aphasia is appraised, the majority of studies constitute low quality evidence according to the CEBM (2009) hierarchy. They are frequently Level 3 or lower. Many global aphasia studies also have significant methodological flaws, and/or do not provide sufficient detail for therapists to replicate in a clinical setting. Nevertheless, it is important to understand what can be learnt from the evidence that is available and this chapter will summarise this literature. It is helpful to highlight at this point that studies of global aphasia have generally sought to answer one of two questions: Either they have sought to establish whether SLT (in a broad sense) can lead to improvements in this population, or they have sought to ascertain whether a particular type of SLT treatment has favourable outcomes.

Can SLT lead to improvements for PwGA?

An important question when considering this question is, "What constitutes SLT?" Historically, SLT intervention was wholly impairment based and focused on restoring the language system. An approach referred to as "language stimulation" (see Schuell et al.,

1964) was often used. Language stimulation is essentially impairment-based therapy involving tasks such as repeating words, repeating phrases, naming pictures, completing phrases, completing word associations, reading in unison, and spelling. Over time and with the World Health Organization's (2001) International Classification of Functioning, Disability and Health framework now embedded into clinical practice, SLT intervention is broader and more holistic. Psychosocial factors, the provision of education, compensatory strategies, and opportunities for social participation are all considered within the intervention process. However, many studies of global aphasia are old and date back to the 1980s prior to this more holistic SLT approach being standard practice. Consequently, most studies of global aphasia have investigated impairment-based/language stimulation approaches and used impairment level outcome measures.

Samples and Lane (1980) reported based on findings from a single case study that improvements can be made in global aphasia, but the trajectory of recovery may be longer than in other aphasia types. Their client improved on multiple subtests of the Porch Index of Communicative Ability (PICA; Porch, 1967) after receiving language stimulation SLT alongside Melodic Intonation Therapy (MIT; Albert, Sparks, & Helm, 1973) twice weekly for three months and then five times a week for three years. This is a considerable amount of intervention and when one looks at the specific scores reported, some changes are very small. PICA overall score improved from 6.1 to 10.51 in the three-year period. Verbal score improved from 2.2 to 6.9 and graphic (writing) score from 6.62 to 8.3. Gesture was the only area to move more markedly from 7.36 to 13.94. From a methodological point of view, this being a single case study limits its usefulness for generalising to other PwGA and the lack of discussion in the paper about if or how the changes were reflected functionally is an important omission. Nevertheless, the study suggests MIT may be a beneficial approach and that gesture may be amenable to treatment in this population.

In a larger study of seven PwGA, Sarno and Levita (1981) also reported positive benefits after SLT. All participants received intervention based on the language stimulation approach (which included some group sessions) three to five times weekly for one year. Their participants were tested at four, eight, 26, and 52 weeks post stroke using the Functional Communication Profile (Sarno, 1969), the BDAE (Goodglass & Kaplan, 1972), the Token Test (De Renzi & Vignolo, 1962) as well as with naming, sentence repetition, and word fluency tasks. They found that all participants improved over the first year. Examples provided were that all participants improved on the Token Test with the level of change varying from 31 to 76 points and all improved in at least three of the other assessments. There are issues with this study in that no control tasks were used and no statistical testing completed. A positive is that whilst not robustly measured, some information is provided about functional communication changes. For example, anecdotal descriptions of an increase in spontaneous speech, increase in the frequency and length of short phrases and sentences, and increased comprehension in social conversation are reported. The improvements were particularly noted to occur in the latter six months post stroke which is in keeping with the finding of Samples and Lane (1980) that PwGA may need SLT for longer than six months.

A similar finding is that of Smania et al. (2010) who detailed a case study of a patient with global aphasia who was tested in language, praxis, and intelligence over a period of 25 years. Their client received SLT intervention for the first two years after stroke, starting with five times a week for the first six months and then three times weekly for 18 months. The content of intervention is not discussed in the paper. The outcome measures were the Milan language examination (MLE; Milan University Neuropsychology Center, 1974), the Token Test (De Renzi & Vignolo, 1962), RCPM (Raven, 1956), and apraxia tests. These were completed at three weeks, two months, six months, one year, two years, three years, ten years, 21 years, and 25 years after stroke. Significant improvements in each language function (comprehension, repetition, reading, naming, and event description) were found over time. The authors analysed the nature of recovery in more detail and found that in the first year after stroke there was significant improvement in comprehension of simple conceptualised tasks measured in the MLE (Milan University Neuropsychology Center, 1974), but recovery of more abstract comprehension measured in the Token Test (De Renzi & Vignolo, 1962) took longer. Repetition improved most during the first year and continued to improve over ten years. Reading and naming abilities emerged between one and three years after stroke and progressively improved, reaching 45% of performance in twenty-five years. Spontaneous speech as measured in their event description task emerged approximately ten years after stroke and then slightly improved over time. The findings support the suggestion of a longer trajectory of recovery in global aphasia and suggest that improvements are possible well after the cessation of SLT. However, as it is a single case study (Level 5 evidence) generalising and drawing conclusions is difficult.

As mentioned earlier, RCTs are considered Level 1 evidence. The only RCT specific to PwGA was conducted by Denes, Perazzolo, Piani, and Piccione (1996). Sixty-three participants were randomly allocated to an experimental group who received daily (intensive) SLT averaging 125 sessions over six months or a control group who received a standard dose of SLT two or three times weekly, averaging 60 sessions over six months. Sessions lasted

45-60 minutes. Importantly, the intervention in this study is described as "ecological." The focus was on using language in a conversational context and total communication, that is using all means of communication (speaking, gesturing, and facial expression). Impairment-based semantic and comprehension tasks which increased in complexity were also carried out. The mean scores on language subtests of the Aachen Aphasia Test (Luzzatti, Willmes, & De Bleser, 1991) for each group were compared statistically after intervention. The authors found more participants in the intensive group made statistically significant improvements after intervention than those in the regular group. However, when the results are unpacked, the differences are quite small. For example, six participants in the intensive group made significant gains in repetition compared with five in the regular group. The only difference that was more substantial was in writing whereby five participants in the intensive group improved compared with one in the regular group. Yet this is a confusing finding because writing was not an area targeted in treatment. A significant problem is that the intervention in this study is not clearly described so it is impossible for a clinician to replicate. Whilst the authors concluded from their findings that PwGA benefit from intensive SLT, the data are more nuanced. The intensive group differed not only by intensity but also by dose (overall number of sessions) so this could partially explain the difference found. Yet despite the enhanced intensity and dose there were still only small differences between the groups, suggesting intensive SLT may not be significantly beneficial in global aphasia. One further issue is that the outcome measure (Aachen Aphasia Test; Luzzatti et al., 1991) is fundamentally a language rather than functional assessment. Given the content of intervention was "ecological" and relatively functional in nature it may not be the most appropriate assessment for effectively capturing the improvements participants may have made. It is possible that more significant differences between the two groups would have been noted had a functional measure been used. In summary, this is the only RCT available on global aphasia. It demonstrates that PwGA can make improvements after SLT but it is unclear from the findings whether the population benefit from increased intensity or overall dose.

In summary, evidence suggests PwGA can make impairment level gains after SLT intervention if offered intensive or prolonged periods of intervention. The degree of such improvement may be small and the functional impact is mostly unknown. The capacity for services to offer the documented intensity and dose of treatment is an issue. In the wider aphasia literature there is increasing evidence about the benefits of Intensive Comprehensive Aphasia Programmes (ICAPs) whereby clients are offered a minimum of three hours of treatment daily over at least two weeks (Rose, Cherney, & Worrall, 2013; Monnelly, Marshall, & Cruice, 2021; Leff et al., 2021). Whilst it is unclear whether PwGA can tolerate or benefit from such programmes, it may be that the doses prescribed in some studies become a possibility in the future if services take up this model of delivery. The limited exploration of functional outcomes after therapy in the previous studies is a significant omission but reflects the clinical focus at the time those research studies were carried out. Within the literature exploring specific interventions for global aphasia there is more discussion of functional outcomes. Studies that have trialled specific interventions with PwGA will be discussed next.

What is the evidence for specific intervention approaches in global aphasia?

Remnant picture books

Remnant books are communication books which contain real items that depict places or events such as tickets, maps, prayer cards, and magazine covers. Ho et al. (2005) compared supported conversation treatment using communication books containing only pictures/ photos with supported conversation treatment using remnant books in two PwGA. The participants were reported to have retained some ability to indicate "yes" and "no" and understand single words in context but could not initiate interactions spontaneously at baseline. Intervention involved the communication partner (a trained SaLT) interacting with the participant using one type of book, asking them at least three open questions and making at least three general comments, followed by a break and then interaction with the other type of book. Participants had sessions daily over five days. Intervention sessions were all recorded. Baseline and post intervention testing involved a five-minute video-recorded unsupported conversation without a communication book. The video recordings were analysed before, during, and after the intervention and coded for number of conversation turns, topic initiations, communication breakdowns, negative affect, no responses, and pointing. The authors found that both types of books facilitated interactions with an increase in topic initiation and pointing after the intervention compared with baseline. A modest advantage for remnant books over picture books was also noted with one participant initiating more topics and both participants demonstrating increased joint attention and pointing with the remnant book.

In summary, the study suggests that use of a communication book is advantageous in global aphasia but remnant books perhaps more so. The study provides lots of detail for clinical replication and can be relatively easily implemented clinically. However, the sample size reduces the quality of the evidence somewhat. The participants in this study were offered intervention daily and it is unclear whether the improvements noted are partially due to this. Future research is needed to establish whether daily intervention is necessary for a positive outcome.

Melodic intonation therapy

Melodic Intonation Therapy (MIT; Albert et al., 1973; Helm-Estabrooks, Albert, & Nicholas, 2014) is a hierarchically structured method of eliciting single words and phrases through musical intonation and exaggerated prosody initially and then normal intonation and prosody later. The method is intended for use with people who have little to no spontaneous speech output and poor repetition in the presence of moderately preserved comprehension. This description is in keeping with severe non-fluent (Broca's) aphasia. However, MIT has been used with PwGA as in the study by Samples and Lane (1980) described earlier in this chapter. Morrow-Odom and Swann (2013) also describe the use of MIT with a client with global aphasia. They delivered MIT alongside cognitive tasks such as symbol cancellation and shape and symbol sequencing to a participant with global aphasia in 32 sessions of 2.5-hour length spread over a seven-week period. Each session involved 90 minutes of MIT with short five-minute breaks in which the cognitive tasks were completed. The authors' explanation for the inclusion of cognitive tasks was to disrupt the potential monotony of the 2.5-hour long sessions and reduce fatigue. The cognitive tasks were non-linguistic and did not include letters or numbers to avoid indirectly training language. After the intervention, the participant was found to have improved in performance on all subtests of the Aphasia Diagnostic Profiles (Helm-Estabrooks, 1992) including the severity standard score. However, the participant's overall aphasia classification did not change, and they persisted with global aphasia. Importantly, functional communication changes were captured using the ASHA-FACS (Frattali et al., 1995) and the communication independence score was found to have increased from 3.81 before the intervention to 4.21 post intervention. This change represents a clinically important improvement with the client requiring moderate to maximal assistance to functionally communicate at baseline (i.e. frequently needing assistance/prompting) then moving to requiring only moderate assistance (i.e. often needing assistance/prompting) after intervention. After intervention, the participant was noted by her husband to be using more gesture in context, counting during card games, and making more spontaneous production attempts. There was no change on the SA-QOL-39 (Hilari et al., 2003) after intervention. Morrow-Odom and Swann (2013) concluded that MIT is a suitable treatment for PwGA, which is consistent with my own clinical experience. However, the authors did not acknowledge the influence the cognitive treatments completed alongside MIT may have indirectly had on outcomes. Further research using MIT with PwGA is required.

Gesture and non-linguistic treatments

Visual Action Therapy (VAT; Helm-Estabrooks et al., 1982) is a non-verbal treatment for global aphasia designed to be conducted as a precursor to communication treatment. It aims to improve communicative intent (desire to communicate) and the ability to relay concepts through gesture. VAT works outside the modality of speech and is non-linguistic, using real objects, pictures, and gestures instead. There are 12 steps in the VAT programme (Helm-Estabrooks et al., 1982; Helm-Estabrooks et al., 2014) which are ordered hierarchically based on level of difficulty from basic tasks involving matching objects and pictures to more advanced tasks requiring understanding of pictures and gestures and production of gestures. One hundred percent success is required at each step before progressing to the next. In a study of eight PwGA, Helm-Estabrooks et al. (1982) found statistically significant improvements in the production of gesture after they received VAT for 30 minutes a day for four to 14 weeks. The exact duration of therapy was dependent on the individual participant's progression through the steps. A benefit is that the intervention is non-verbal and thus easily accessible to PwGA. Furthermore, because no verbal instructions are provided, the client has to use non-verbal reasoning and problem-solving skills to understand task requirements – skills which are highly relevant to functional communication. The study by Helm-Estabrooks et al. (1982) constitutes Level 3 evidence but has flaws due to no control task being offered to clients. The intervention is however clearly described and can easily be replicated clinically. The only issue SaLTs may find is that replicating the daily intervention used in the study may be difficult in their clinical settings. In clinical practice I have used VAT with less intensive delivery (such as twice or three times weekly due to service constraints) and still had favourable outcomes.

One interesting finding from the study of VAT is that despite the intervention being non-linguistic and using no verbal or written words, statistically significant improvement in auditory comprehension was observed after the intervention. There was also a trend towards significant improvement in reading comprehension despite no written language tasks being used. The mechanism for these indirect improvements is difficult to unpack but suggests that non-verbal intervention and/or training cognitive skills either contributes to language gains or provides clients with the skills to more accurately complete language assessments and demonstrate their potential. A similar finding was recently demonstrated in my unpublished study of six PwGA (Adjei-Nicol, 2020) whereby a non-linguistic cognitive treatment programme involving sessions conducted non-verbally led to indirect improvements in auditory comprehension for some participants. Non-linguistic interventions are not yet commonplace in SLT but show promise as an approach.

Although Helm-Estabrooks et al. (1982) did not measure functional communication changes after VAT, I have found this intervention often leads to functional improvements in gesture comprehension and on occasion gesture production also. VAT primarily aims to teach gesture but the technique indirectly also targets selective attention, visual semantics, visual-perceptual skills, and problem-solving skills. As has been discussed throughout this book, cognitive skills are essential for successful functional communication. Therefore, it may be that the indirect training of underlying cognitive skills is responsible for the functional gains I have seen in clinical practice.

In summary, VAT is an intervention easily accessible to PwGA that can improve gestural comprehension and production. In some cases, improvements can generalise to functional gains in gesture and indirect gains in auditory comprehension. The findings from VAT suggest an advantage for treating cognitive skills and using non-verbal treatments with this population.

Non-verbal communication

Total communication is an approach which aims to facilitate communication using any modality possible (speech, writing, drawing, facial expression, pointing, using pictures or objects). In some cases, it is referred to as "multimodal therapy." In a survey conducted with UK-based SaLTs working with PwGA (Adjei, 2015; Adjei-Nicol, 2020), 95% of respondents reported using a total communication approach with clients. Although widely used in SLT, there is very little literature about its efficacy as a treatment for aphasia and no consensus as to what total communication/multimodal therapy should entail.

One intervention often used to train clients in total communication is Promoting Aphasics' Communicative Effectiveness (PACE; Davis & Wilcox, 1981, 1985). PACE is a barrier task that emphasises semi-natural communication. It involves the SaLT and PwA taking turns to give and receive messages. The sender must convey the information portrayed on a picture card to the receiver (who cannot see it) using any modality available to them (consistent with total communication). The receiver must then guess what is relayed in the picture. Part of the intervention involves the receiver providing feedback to the sender on how successful they have been at conveying the message. One benefit of PACE is the way it mimics real-life communication in that one person (the receiver) genuinely does not know the content of the other person's card and has to guess. This is comparable to real-life situations in which the communication partner often does not know the message and is reliant on guesswork. PACE also allows for the SaLT to play an active role in therapy: rather than the client always being the sender and having to relay a message, sometimes it is the therapist doing so. Potentially, depending on the ability of the client, the intervention may also involve the SaLT receiving feedback from the client on how well they have conveyed the picture. This can be empowering for the client and provides some balance in the therapeutic relationship. This is an aspect of therapy that is very difficult to achieve when working with clients with severe impairments who are often reliant on the SaLT for feedback.

In global aphasia, PACE has never been investigated as an individual therapy but has been offered in combination with other approaches. For example, Lawson and Fawcus (1999) described a client with global aphasia who received PACE alongside total communication group therapy focused on miming, drawing, reading, and writing. The intervention was provided twice a week for eight months and gains were reported in the use of gesture, drawing, and mime in real-life situations.

Ward-Lonergan and Nicholas (1995) delivered PACE alongside an extensive range of other interventions. The authors adapted PACE by encouraging the client to focus on one modality (drawing). In addition to PACE, their client received VAT, gesture therapy, and drawing therapy over the course of three years. The client was reported to have improved from a score of 27 to 39 (50th to 95th percentile for PwGA) on the Boston Assessment of Severe Aphasia (Helm-Estabrooks, Ramsberger, Morgan, & Nicholas, 1989). Whilst no gains in verbal output were found, functional improvements were noted. For example, drawings were found to be more recognisable as judged by an independent assessor and the participant was reportedly using spontaneous gestures and some writing in conjunction with drawing when communicating. Given the breadth of intervention provided, it is not possible to know which element(s) are most relevant to the positive improvements or what role PACE specifically played in the overall outcome. Ward-Lonergan and Nicholas (1995) suggest the client's motivation, good recall for life events, good spatial orientation and attention to detail may have aided response to treatment and particularly the drawing therapies. Once again this is a single case study with no control task, so only cautious interpretation of findings is possible. The duration of intervention is also not viable in most contexts. Like Ward-Lonergan and Nicholas (1995) I also often modify PACE and encourage clients to use one specific modality to relay their message rather than any or all means. This is because the severe semantic deficits PwGA often have may preclude their ability to access semantic representations in multiple different modalities. Another challenge for clients when total communication is attempted as part of PACE is that their cognitive difficulties prevent them switching between communication modalities easily.

Augmentative and alternative communication (AAC)

"Augmentative and alternative communication" is a term used to describe methods, devices, or strategies that enable people to compensate for communication challenges. AAC can be divided into categories of "aided" or "unaided" and "no tech," "low tech," or "high tech." Unaided AAC refers to methods that do not require a physical aid or tool, whereas aided AAC does. No tech AAC requires no materials other than one's body such as head nodding/ shaking, thumbs up/down, miming, and iconic gesture. Low tech AAC typically involves paper-based, static displays such as Yes/No charts, picture communication books, and charts. High tech AAC on the other hand usually involves power or rechargeable battery-operated devices and voice output.

In clinical practice no tech/low tech AAC such as gesture, objects, picture communication charts, and communication books are more frequently used with PwGA than high tech AAC. Usually, the aim of AAC in global aphasia is to enable clients to express single concepts relevant to functional needs. Attempts to teach PwGA to use high tech systems for more complex messages or abstract semiotic (symbol) systems have not been particularly successful as illustrated by the following studies.

C-VIC is a computerised communication system using abstract symbols to represent nouns, verbs, and thematic relationships. McCall et al. (2000) taught this system to a client with chronic global aphasia over a three-year period, delivering intervention three times a week. They found that the client did develop the ability to construct basic sentences using the system. However, this did not generalise to everyday contexts. Koul, Corwin, and Hayes (2004) found that the two participants with global aphasia in their study were unable to learn the use of a computer-based symbol communication system called GUS. Like C-VIC, GUS uses abstract symbols to represent various parts of language, and the therapy programme involves progressing through hierarchically ordered tasks. In the basic level, clients are taught to access the software using a touch screen, understand that the symbols are hierarchically organised over several screens, and move across symbol screens. To progress to the next level, clients must demonstrate the ability to locate and identify symbols from an auditory instruction with 100% accuracy. The more complex level within the treatment programme required clients to use GUS to produce sentences of increasing grammatical complexity with the symbols they had identified in the first phase. The authors found that participants with global aphasia could not meet the 100% accuracy criterion of Level 1 and were therefore unable to progress beyond the most basic level. In contrast, those with severe (Broca's) aphasia performed better, with some able to produce sentences of varying complexity using the system. The abstract nature of these semiotic symbols is likely a significant contributory factor to the challenges PwGA have with these systems. Furthermore, the linguistic abilities of most PwGA will hinder their ability to generate sentence level messages. Generally, high tech AAC that use pictures/photographs and single concept ideas or messages will be most beneficial for PwGA.

Conversation-based approaches

The only study of conversation-based therapy specific to global aphasia is a single case study completed by Basso (2010). Intervention known as "natural conversation" was delivered to a client with global aphasia for two hours daily for an initial three-month period and then for one hour daily for six months. The exact content of the natural conversation intervention is not described in detail in the paper. The rationale provided for this is that the intervention is focused on the interaction between the client and the therapist rather than intervention tasks. However, some helpful suggestions are provided on how to engage in conversation with PwGA, including making good eye contact, being explicit about speech tasks by making statements such as "I am going to ask you a question" prior to asking one, being explicit when changing topic, and avoiding asking questions one already knows the answer to (a concept sometimes referred to as asking "test questions"). After conversation treatment the client made gains in object naming which reportedly improved by 50% and sentence production which improved by 40%. Functional improvements were also reported by the SaLT and the participant's wife in terms of the client showing more interest in his surroundings and being more capable of engaging in a supported conversation. Aside from the obvious limitations of this being a single case study, other issues are that information on the language outcome measure used is not provided and the methodology did not involve use of a control measure. Despite the positive outcomes described in this particular case study, my clinical observations suggest conversational approaches are challenging with PwGA unless they are slightly higher level with a presentation bordering with severe aphasia. Indeed, this is consistent with descriptions in the literature. No study has explored communication partner training specifically for PwGA. Kagan (1999) has described successful use of an approach called Supported Conversations for Adults with Aphasia (SCA) with PwSA and documented that those who benefit most from this approach have relatively good comprehension and some ability to indicate "yes" and "no" consistently. The approach involves family and carers being trained to use strategies that enable the client to engage in conversation. Kagan suggests that clients who have difficulty indicating "yes" and "no" may require intervention to aid readiness for supported conversation treatment. The content of such intervention is not discussed but I presume this to involve tasks aimed at improving comprehension and ability to provide a yes/no response. Kagan concludes that if "readiness" intervention is unsuccessful, then supported conversation as an approach is not suitable for the client. There are however ways that conversation-based approaches can be adapted for use with PwGA. This will be discussed in Chapter 5.

Chapter summary

In summary, few intervention studies have included PwGA. Those that have are more than a decade old, have not demonstrated functional gains, or have methodological flaws constituting low quality evidence. The evidence that does exist suggests traditional language-based SLT alone is unlikely to lead to functional gains but in high doses may lead to impairment level gains. Available evidence suggests PwGA may benefit from approaches such as VAT (Helm-Estabrooks et al., 1982), PACE (Davis & Wilcox, 1981, 1985), non-linguistic cognitive focused treatment (Adjei-Nicol, 2020), and using non-verbal communication/AAC such as gesture, drawing, and communication books.

5

INTERVENTION IN CLINICAL PRACTICE

Introduction

Given the limited research evidence available on intervention in global aphasia, it is necessary to utilise clinical experience and expertise to support evidence-based practice. This chapter is divided into two sections. Part 1 will describe a range of direct intervention approaches and tasks that I have successfully used with PwGA. The three case studies discussed earlier in this book will be used as a framework to illustrate the different tasks and approaches that may be suitable for clients with varying degrees of severity. Part 2 will describe indirect therapy approaches that can be used to in place of or to complement direct treatment.

Part 1: direct intervention

The profiles of three PwGA were presented in Chapter 1 and demonstrated that there are varying levels of cognitive impairment and functional communication abilities in those with global aphasia. Case Study 1 described Mrs M who had profound linguistic and cognitive impairments and little to no functional communication abilities. Case Study 2 described Mr B who had severe linguistic impairments, moderate cognitive impairments, and some limited functional communication skills. Case Study 3 described Mr P who had some limited residual language, somewhat spared cognitive skills, and relatively good functional communication abilities. This section will take each of these clients in turn and detail the specific interventions that were carried out with them as well as other tasks that may be suitable for clients at a similar level.

Case study 1: Mrs M

Mrs M has profound aphasia, limb apraxia, and little to no functional communication abilities. She is unable to complete any assessment due to her passiveness and limited

DOI: 10.4324/9781003184522-5

initiation. She is unable to use a basic communication chart, gesture, drawing, or pointing to objects to communicate and has limited attention skills:

Mrs M's intervention goals were to be able to do as follows:

- Engage in looking at a family photo album with her husband for ten minutes, showing signs of joint focus and understanding of the activity by turning pages and scanning photos
- Use a Yes/No chart to respond to basic verification questions within structured activities
- Engage in a picture sorting task with her daughter on three occasions, showing signs of turn taking and correctly sorting at least half of the pictures by category

In terms of non-linguistic cognitive interventions needed for Mrs M, her case study (see Chapter 1) suggests she has a range of difficulties alongside her aphasia. These include difficulties with executive functioning, basic social communication, visual perception, and non-verbal semantics (difficulties in accessing meanings from pictures, objects, and gestures). I have found that clients who present with both severe cognitive and severe linguistic difficulties benefit greatly from non-verbal and non-linguistic treatment approaches. Non-verbal treatment involves limiting and if possible completely removing the use of verbal language from sessions. Instead, instructions and feedback are provided through demonstration and gesture. The client's responses during sessions are also intended to be non-verbal, for example pointing or gesture. Non-linguistic treatment involves removing all language (use of spoken or written words) from tasks and focusing on cognitive skills such as visual perception or attention instead. These skills underpin communication and the SLT process. In my experience, cognitive treatment even when delivered without any linguistic focus can lead to improvement in functional communication and/or engagement in SLT. For some clients once cognitive skills have somewhat improved, it may be appropriate to proceed with more traditional SLT approaches/tasks that involve verbal instructions and use of spoken and written words. However, for others who are profoundly impaired, linguistic options may never become viable. Some examples of non-linguistic tasks follow.

Non-Linguistic tasks

Basic card games

Card games are a useful way to develop joint focus and turn-taking skills. The SaLT has a pile of cards and takes a card from this pile and places it on the table (between themselves and the client) to start a new pile. Using gesture, facial expression, and some limited spoken language (e.g. "your turn"), the client is encouraged to also take a card from the original pile and place it in the new pile started by the therapist. The SaLT and the client should do this in turns, with the goal that the client is jointly focusing on the task at hand, taking their turn appropriately, and initiating placing the card on the pile without prompting. At this level what is on the card is irrelevant, and there is no requirement to match cards. The client is simply learning to (1) follow the lead of the SLT without verbal instruction, (2) take turns in a task, and (3) carry out the same behaviour repetitively – all skills relevant to SLT and basic communication. Initially, and especially with those with limb apraxia, the SaLT may need to take the client's hand to support them to initiate taking a card. In some cases the SaLT may need to continue with the physical assistance and help the client place the card down. Over time this support should gradually be withdrawn.

Although there is no requirement to match cards in this instance, it is still best to keep the card set as simple as possible. Rather than use a deck of playing cards, one could use more simplistic matching cards such as those often used with children with objects or shapes on them. It is important however to consider whether such cards are too childish and inappropriate for the adult client. Alternatively, object picture cards such as the "Everyday Objects" deck (Speechmark, 2012) found widely in SLT can be used.

Visual attention tasks

Visual attention tasks can be useful for improving a client's ability to attend to and scan between visual stimuli. One task is for the SaLT to move objects in the client's line of vision, with the aim being for the client to visually follow the object. This type of task is often used in a neurological examination or in assessments of clients in prolonged disorders of consciousness. However, the key factor in doing this as a therapy task rather than as an assessment is to provide support if needed. It is not unusual for me to be moving an object in the client's line of vision with one arm while using my other arm to physically move the client's head to demonstrate the need to track and look at the target. After providing maximal physical prompts initially, these can gradually be removed.

I have found it easier to practice visual attention tasks using a computer with an item moving across the screen in different directions than physical objects as this allows more freedom for providing physical prompts. One way to quickly create a computerised version of a visual tracking task is to use Microsoft PowerPoint. Options such as "Float In" or "Fly In" on the Animation Pane in PowerPoint allow items (e.g. an image of an object) to move across a slide. By selecting "Effect Options" the direction you wish the item to move across the slide can be adjusted (e.g. from bottom left or from top left) and the duration of the movement set. Once the slide is presented as slideshow, the picture will move across the screen in the direction set. Multiple slides can be created with pictures set to move in different directions across the screen. Support during the training of this skill might again include helping the client to move their head in the direction of the moving item or the SaLT following the item with their finger and prompting the client to focus on where they are pointing.

A variation of the visual scanning task is for the client to practice shifting their gaze from one item to another. I find this task to be highly relevant to functional communication, arguably more so than visual tracking. In this case the client is required to look *between* two options such as two images or two real objects. This can be done in two ways. The first is to hold an item in one position, such as in your left hand, and then ask the client to look at it. Once they have done so, a new item is presented in a different position, such as on the right side or above or below the original target. At the same time as presenting this new item the SaLT must simultaneously remove the initial item from the client's view. The goal is for the client to shift the focus of their gaze to this new location. This is sometimes referred to as "shifting gaze without competition." That is, the client is learning to look to a new target when the initial target is no longer in their vision. The issue for many clients initially with this task is not that they fail to look to the new target but do so after a significant delay or only after much prompting. This task is a useful stepping-stone towards the more functionally relevant method of "shifting gaze *with* competition." In this task, the SaLT once again starts by presenting an item in one position, and once the client looks at it, the SaLT should then present a second item in a different position such as above, below, or to the right or left of the original. However, this time the initial item is not removed. The client must learn to shift their gaze to the new item whilst the original item is still present. The ability to do this is highly relevant to functional situations in which clients are asked to make a choice between pictures or objects with all the stimuli remaining in position. In these gaze shift tasks, there is no requirement to recognise or gain meaning from the stimuli. The client is merely asked to look between the stimuli. Again, it is possible to create a task like this in PowerPoint, this time using the "Appear" option in the animation pane and manipulating the positions in which the target image appears.

In some cases, it is helpful if the targets used in visual attention tasks are not meaningful objects or pictures. It is possible that by using meaningful items the client allocates some of their attention to attempting to recognise the item and accessing their semantic system. This may lead to less attention being allocated to the primary goal of the task which is to visually attend to stimuli and an overall poor performance. A simple black or coloured circle on a piece of paper (or on a screen) can mitigate for this issue. On the other hand, some clients may find a meaningless target such as this uninteresting and dull and therefore not engage with the task. In such cases the therapist could consider using pictures but must exercise caution when interpreting the client's performance. If pictures are to be used, items that can actually fly/move as targets, such as a bird, bee, aeroplane, or butterfly, may be more meaningful options.

A useful resource when considering visual tracking and gaze shift abilities is the eye-pointing classification scale (UCL, 2020). This scale was designed as a way for professionals and families to describe looking behaviours in children with cerebral palsy (Clarke et al., 2022). Whilst the tool cannot be used to classify the behaviours of PwGA, the descriptions of different types of looking behaviours are extremely helpful when designing and evaluating visual attention tasks.

Matching tasks

Playing a basic Snap card game whereby the card set used contains matching pairs is another non-linguistic task useful for clients at Mrs M's level. This can be commenced once clients are proficient at the basic card game described earlier. As outlined then, the SaLT has a pile of cards and takes a card from this pile and places it on the table (between themselves and the client) to start a new pile. Using gesture, facial expression, and some limited language (such as "your turn," "yes," "no"), the clinician should demonstrate that some cards are the same and some cards are not the same/different. I often bring in the concept of "yes" and "no" at this point, saying "yes" to highlight cards that match and "no" when cards do not. The SaLT and client should take turns as before, taking a card from the original pile and placing it on the new pile, this time looking out for when cards match. Each time that cards do not match I emphasise this by saying "no" and using the thumbs down gesture. When I have or the client has cards that do match I say "yes" and give a thumbs up. The client may require significant cues and prompts to recognise the matching of the cards. Depending on the client's level of comprehension, the complexity of the task can be increased to include the client and SLT each having their own individual pile or adding the requirement to verbally say "snap" when two cards match.

Matching tasks can be extended to involve gaze shifting practice also. The client can be given a target object or image and asked to match it to an identical item from an array of objects or pictures. To do this successfully requires the client to employ skills developed in the previously mentioned visual attention tasks of shifting gaze between items when there are competing targets. A further task might be to match objects to pictures or match pictures to objects. This requires clients to be able to identify similarities despite the object being three-dimensional and the picture two-dimensional.

Mrs M initially found matching objects to pictures and pictures to objects difficult. In such cases it can be useful to consider tracing around objects as a task (see Step 1 within the VAT programme; Helm-Estabrooks et al., 1982). Tracing objects (with support if needed) and matching the line drawing to the original object can help clients understand that a physical three-dimensional object can be represented as a two-dimensional line drawing/image. This skill is something clinicians can take for granted but I have known many clients to require this to be explicitly taught before they can move on to any tasks which use pictures as stimuli.

The Language Activity Resource Kit 2 (LARK-2; Dressler, 2005) is a very useful resource to have available for carrying out the aforementioned matching tasks in a busy clinical setting where there is limited time to find matching pictures or produce individualised items. It contains two sets of real objects, colour photographs, line drawings, and written words depicting the same everyday items which the clinician can use freely to practice tasks such as object matching, object-picture matching, verbal or written word to picture matching, gesture to picture matching, gesture production, and many other tasks. In the manual, Dressler (2005) proposes that the tool can be used to help PwGA learn alternative methods for communication.

Throughout all the previously mentioned tasks, the clinician should try not to verbally explain tasks and instead use only demonstration (multiple times if necessary), exaggerated facial expressions, and gesture to illustrate when items match or not. The concepts "yes" and "no" may however be used verbally or with a Yes/No chart within the task. In the same way, clients should be encouraged to observe the SaLT's demonstrations and interpret their facial expressions and gestures to understand the task. This builds their problem-solving and non-verbal communication skills. Initially, the client may be presented with only two items to choose from in matching tasks, but with increasing accuracy of performance the number of items in the array might be increased.

Basic selective attention tasks

When we present a choice of objects/pictures to a client there is a need for them to disregard the irrelevant option and focus on the target. This requires selective attention abilities. The need to selectively attend to a target is a pre-requisite for SLT assessments, intervention tasks, and functional communication situations, as has been detailed in Chapter 2, but it is rarely considered in SLT. In my opinion it is the most important area to target in clients presenting with significant cognitive overlay to their aphasia as is the case for Mrs M.

A task for developing this skill is to present the client with a target picture and keep this in the client's line of vision. The client should be instructed through gesture, facial expression, and demonstration that they will be shown a variety of pictures (one at a time) but they are to respond only when the picture shown is the same as their target. They are not to respond when the picture is of something else (a distractor picture). The SaLT should have access to a number of copies of the target picture mixed in with other pictures. Initially, when practicing the task, the distractors should not be semantically connected to the target but distant distractors. A suitable way for the client to respond when they see the target should be determined. This could be that they raise their hand, press a switch, tap the table, or indicate "yes." The SaLT then presents one picture at a time. These will be randomly ordered distractor or target pictures. The SaLT should demonstrate the task a few times, emphasising that the client should not respond to the irrelevant pictures but only to the pictures which are identical to their target. This task can appear relatively straightforward, especially when the target picture remains in the client's view throughout the task. However, it is common for PwGA to make errors such as responding to irrelevant pictures, not responding when the target is shown, or perseverating and responding to all pictures. This highlights the types of issues they have functionally when presented with a choice of two objects or a communication chart and are asked to make a selection. They may not be able to selectively attend to the relevant item they want and therefore fail to make a selection, point to an item they do not want or, in many cases, point to all options. When clients make errors in this selective attention task, they should be corrected and reminded of the target and task requirements. During the session, the target picture can be changed intermittently for variety and to place a further demand on cognition by requiring the client to switch their focus to a new target. Complexity can also be increased by including more semantically related distractors within the set or increasing the demand on WM by showing the target initially but then removing it. During the process of completing this intervention task, SaLTs should carefully monitor the types of errors clients make. If semantically related distractors are used, there may be occasions when overall accuracy remains poor but the error pattern reflects some progress. For example, if clients move from initially demonstrating no understanding of the task (e.g. by responding to all stimuli including unrelated distractors) to later responding more discretely ignoring unrelated distractors but sometimes incorrectly responding to semantic distractors, then even though accuracy remains low, there is evidence of improvement in selective attention skills.

Basic non-verbal semantic tasks

The previously mentioned matching and selective attention tasks do not necessarily require clients to understand what the objects or pictures are. It is possible to perform the task accurately merely by recognising the visual similarities. The next step is to build object semantic skills and include within the task a requirement to interpret the object and understand its meaning. A task I often do first is what I call "matching to non-identical exemplars." Objects or pictures can be used but this time the two objects must not be identical; instead, they should be different examples of the same item. For example, the client will be provided with a picture of a blue mug and asked to choose from an array the picture it matches with. In this case, rather than the target being an identical blue mug, the target will still be a mug but differ in colour, size, or shape. To successfully complete the task, the client must recognise similarities in shape, visual features, and the meaning/use of the object in the pictures. Once again, despite seeming to be a relatively simple task, this can be challenging for clients with more severe forms of global aphasia. Many only recognise items as the same when they are identical and fail to draw out commonalities (often due to underlying semantic issues).

Through feedback, the SaLT can help highlight commonalities to the client. This can be done by tracing around objects/pictures to highlight visual similarities in shape or the SaLT gesturing the use of the object and highlighting that the gestures and therefore the use is the same for both items. It is often easier to do this task using real objects than pictures, as it is relatively easy to find two non-identical objects such as pens or mugs around the ward or client's home compared with having to source two non-identical pictures of the same item.

A digital version of this task can be found within the Cuespeak (Cuespeak Ltd, 2022) app for PwA. This app contains a huge variety of speech and language tasks and SaLTs can set up tailored programmes to suit the particular level and goals of an individual client. Tasks and items are regularly updated. In the non-verbal matching task within this app, clients must match non-identical examples of the same item or scenario. There are basic items involving non-identical object photos and more complex scenarios. One example is a target photo of an elderly gentleman sitting at a table inside a café. The client must select from an array of four the photo that depicts a similar scenario. In this example the correct response would be to select the photo of a couple sitting at a table in a different café.

Categorising (sorting) objects or pictures by semantic category can be used to further progress non-verbal semantic skills. In this task, two pictures should be set up as the target categories and the client required to place pictures they are given with the corresponding category. To take the categories of food and drink as an example, the client is shown a picture of glass of water to represent the category of drink and this picture placed on one side within the client's visual field. The client is then shown a picture of bread to represent the category of food and this picture placed on the opposite side of the drink picture to represent the alternative category. For demonstration purposes, the SaLT should show the client that the requirement is to place each picture they are presented with on the pile corresponding to the category it belongs to. After demonstrating the task with two items, the client should be presented with one picture at a time belonging to either category in a random order and asked to place it on the corresponding pile. Depending on the severity of the clients' semantic impairments, it may be helpful to use broad and more distantly related categories first before moving on to closer categories such as in the example of food and drink. Wherever possible, categories relevant to the individual client should be used and items selected familiar and appropriate to the client's cultural background and contexts. Some categories I used with Mrs M are as follows:

- Food
- Drink
- Animals
- Clothing
- Furniture
- Transport
- Family
- Friends

Auditory semantic tasks are also beneficial to complete. I commonly include a task requiring clients to match an environmental sound to a picture from an array. For example, the client might listen to the sound of a dog barking or a car engine starting and match it to a picture of these items. To enhance functional communication, it is necessary to enable clients both to take meaning from sounds in their environment and to differentiate background environmental noise from linguistic stimuli. In my study of the effect of a non-linguistic cognitive intervention programme on functional communication (Adjei-Nicol, 2020), the sound to picture matching task was one of six tasks found to be most relevant to positive outcomes. Speechmark (2004a, 2004b) resources are helpful for this task and contain a CD with indoor or outdoor environmental sounds and colour photographs to match these. The aforementioned Cuespeak app (Cuespeak Ltd, 2022) also contains a sound to picture matching task.

Developing yes/no consistency

Developing the ability to differentiate between the concepts "yes" and "no" is an important foundation communication skill. For a client at Mrs M's level, I would tend to commence work on these concepts through same/different matching tasks and use of a Yes/No chart. Depending on the client's background and comprehension abilities the Yes/No chart would use a tick and a cross, or a thumbs up and a thumbs down or, in rarer cases, happy face and sad face emojis. I have often seen therapists present multiple options for each concept on the same chart. For example, a cross, a thumbs down, and the written word "no" on the same chart. For many PwGA this is likely to increase attentional demands and cause them more confusion so one concept for "yes" and "no" on the chart is preferable as is avoidance of written words. For clients with visual neglect, it can also be helpful to present the options vertically rather than horizontally (see Figure 5.1 for an example). To strengthen the difference between symbols I often use different colours.

Using the identical object/picture matching task described earlier as a framework, the SaLT can randomly either present the client with two identical objects/pictures or two

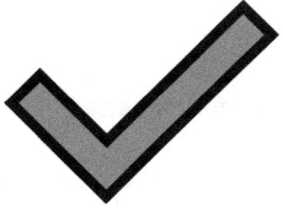

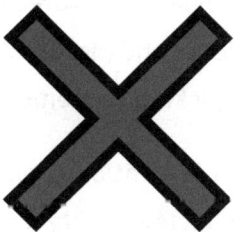

Figure 5.1 Example of a vertical yes/no chart

different objects/pictures. The SaLT then uses the Yes/No chart to demonstrate pointing to the symbol depicting "yes" when the two items match and "no" when they do not. In this task simultaneously verbally saying "yes" and "no" can be useful. After demonstration, the SaLT should continue to randomly present the client with either two identical or non-identical items and provide them with the opportunity to point to "yes" or "no" on the chart as to whether they match. Feedback and further demonstrations should be provided when needed. The task can be extended as client performance improves, for example by completing with the non-identical matching task described earlier or gesture verification. An example of a gesture verification task is the therapist placing one object in front of the client and then producing a gesture that is either congruent or incongruent with the object. The client should use the Yes/No chart to identify whether the gesture matches the object or not.

It is of course perfectly possible to practice yes/no with single word verification tasks, for example showing the client an object (such as a key) and giving a verbal label for the item that is either correct or incorrect ("Is this an apple?"). The client must then point to the Yes/No chart to indicate whether the auditory word is the correct label for the target picture or not. However, given the linguistic impairments of some clients this is often too challenging.

Functional practice and promoting generalisation

By the end of nine weeks of therapy twice a week using the aforementioned tasks, Mrs M had improved in her ability to do the following:

- Share focus with the SaLT
- Take turns in an activity
- Understand basic facial expressions that indicate when something is correct/incorrect
- Understand the concept of same/different
- Understand the concept of yes/no within the context of same/different
- Recognise a selection of objects/pictures
- Understand the meanings of the objects/pictures that have been targeted in therapy
- Scan and shift gaze between objects and pictures
- Initiate pointing to, selecting, or picking up items

As these skills directly linked to her intervention goals so these were achieved. In addition functional changes were noted in Mrs M's ability to look between choices and make a selection by pointing when presented with two objects or pictures, scan through pictures or videos on a tablet and make a selection, and play board games with family with support.

There are cases where targeted functional practice is required before generalisation occurs. In such instances, time might be spent in sessions looking through family photo albums or a magazine of interest and the client encouraged to turn pages independently, scan the page, indicate something of interest, and answer yes/no questions using their communication chart. I frequently include an element of surprise or error in activities to build in some basic problem solving not dissimilar to the suggestions described when detailing functional assessment in Chapter 3. This might be providing incorrect comments/ information when looking through photos such as "Is that your mother?" when it is not or placing cards or a magazine upside down or out of reach. I give the client time to see whether they recognise the issue or try to initiate communicating or resolving the problem. If they do not, I might prompt with an open question or gesture and if still no attempt, highlight the error to the client using basic language and gesture. This can build initiation skills in clients who are very passive by providing them with a reason to need to communicate. In real-life communication contexts, communication is not always straightforward or predictable; indeed, communication around expressing basic needs requires clients to first recognise a problem such as being thirsty or needing the toilet and to then know that the solution is to point to a specific picture or gain someone's attention. Embedding problems, mistakes, and the need to initiate communication within therapy sessions is critical to enhancing underlying skills for successful functional communication.

Joint sessions with family

Non-verbal communication has been a key component to much of the intervention discussed thus far. Ideally, similar strategies should be employed by family to ensure consistency and enable successful communication outside of therapy sessions. Many relatives are initially hesitant about non-verbal treatments and fear that this may hinder the client's potential to improve or use verbal communication. As discussed in Chapter 3 education about global aphasia and SLT early in the client's journey can prevent issues later with compliance and acceptance. Active demonstration is also important by including family in treatment sessions, demonstrating how non-verbal communication can be used effectively and providing family with ideas of how to engage their loved one in activities. Through being active participants and observing some of the benefits, relatives are often more accepting of non-verbal communication. One of the particular challenges working with relatives is developing their ability to limit speech in their interactions. It does not come easily or naturally to many, especially when they have been used to communicating verbally with their loved one. There have been occasions when I have provided relatives with direct sessions or training practicing conveying a message non-verbally or with only a few key words. I also encourage relatives to incorporate an element of surprise within their daily routine to enhance problem solving and initiation abilities. This could be providing the client with no cutlery at a mealtime so there is a need to make a request or after the client makes a choice of drink, "mistakenly" providing the option they did not choose. Often family inadvertently limit communicative attempts for their loved one by following a consistent routine or always anticipating their needs and education about how this may be unhelpful at times is required.

Measuring gains

The main outcome of treatment was Mrs M achieving her goals. However, at the end of treatment she was also re-assessed formally and informally with traditional SLT tasks and assessments that use language. Of note was that after intervention, Mrs M was able to attempt many of the assessments tasks that she could not do at baseline, for example she was able to attempt the spoken word comprehension subtest of the CAT (Swinburn et al., 2004). Mrs M provided no responses at baseline in informal assessment tasks and did not demonstrate scanning or gaze shifting. After intervention, she attempted the entire subtest and provided accurate responses for two targets. Whilst this is a significantly low score, the fact that Mrs M could carry out the assessment is a clinically significant change. As discussed in Chapter 4 when detailing the outcomes of VAT (Helm-Estabrooks et al., 1982), it is possible that improvement in cognitive skills allows clients to understand task requirements and participate in assessment and intervention tasks. Where clients do show such gains they could be offered an opportunity to receive more traditional SLT intervention focused on language. Often with foundation cognitive and communication skills in place clients show increased benefit from SLT.

Case study 2: Mr B

As outlined in Chapters 1 and 3, Mr B has some basic cognitive and functional communication abilities. For example, he is aware of the routine within his care home, can find his way around in his wheelchair, and make choices between two options in function by pointing. Mr B attempts to communicate verbally and non-verbally but produces neologisms and vague gestures and does not always understand what is said to him. His non-verbal "yes" and "no" responses are inconsistent and beyond making choices in specific functional contexts he is unable to use a communication chart or use other forms of non-verbal communication meaningfully.

Mr B's intervention goals were to be able to do the following:

- Express feelings (happy, sad, bored, tired) and ten basic needs (including drink, toilet, go out, bed) using a communication book containing two pictorial options per page

- Use a Yes/No chart to respond to questions about his day in supported conversations
- Recognise and produce five gestures relevant to his daily routine and needs within appropriate contexts

As Mr B is demonstrating some underlying competence in cognitive skills relevant to communication (such as problem solving, initiation, choice making, and basic semantics) he would benefit from a combination of verbal and non-verbal treatment. However, his profile and difficulties suggest that semantic skills need to be enhanced further to include understanding and using gesture, understanding pictures, and understanding and using "yes" and "no." Clients at Mr B's level usually benefit from some verbal language being used in sessions and do not require completely non-linguistic or non-verbal sessions. However, keeping language to single words and short phrases with key words emphasised is usually best.

Moderate level selective attention tasks

The more advanced variations of the selective attention task described with Mrs M earlier were used with Mr B. This involved using closely related (semantic) distractors and then in later sessions, removing the target from Mr B's sight during the task to place additional demands on WM.

A further selective attention task was used to enhance skills relevant to using a communication chart. Mr B was provided with a ten-picture communication chart whilst the SaLT had 20 individual pictures, ten of which were identical to pictures on the communication chart and ten of which were not present on the chart (distractors). The task requires the SaLT to present one picture from the set of individual pictures at a time in a random order and for the client to scan their chart and identify whether the picture matches any on there. The task involves scanning an array of pictures and disregarding irrelevant items or distractor pictures, all skills relevant to functional use of a communication chart. Complexity can be increased by increasing the number of items on the communication chart so that additional scanning is required or providing distractor items which are semantically linked to items on the chart.

Moderate level non-verbal semantic tasks

Category sorting was used with Mr B in a similar way to that described for Mrs M. However, due to his slightly more advanced semantic abilities at baseline, categories used were semantically related such as fruits versus vegetables, bedroom versus kitchen furniture, hot food versus snacks, hot drinks versus cold drinks, alcoholic drinks versus soft drinks, and indoor versus outdoor clothes. Wherever possible, items and categories should be relevant to the client's contexts and personalised.

"Odd one out" tasks are excellent for developing non-verbal semantic skills. Clients must scan an array and decide which item does not have a similar meaning or use to the others. For Mr B, three options were provided initially with one being unrelated to the other two (see Figure 5.2) but over time the number initially provided increased. Usually, I present the set of pictures in a horizontal row in front of the client and demonstrate the task two or three times using basic language such as "yes," "no," "good," and "wrong" and a basic explanation of why an item is odd. In the case of the example shown in Figure 5.2 I would say "not for eating". It is possible to do this task non-verbally if needed, using only facial expression and gesture to highlight the odd picture and not necessarily refer to why the picture is incorrect. The SaLT should consider whether a distantly related target as in Figure 5.2 is appropriate or whether the client is best challenged with a target that is semantically related to other items as in Figure 5.3. This very much depends on the client's semantic abilities at baseline.

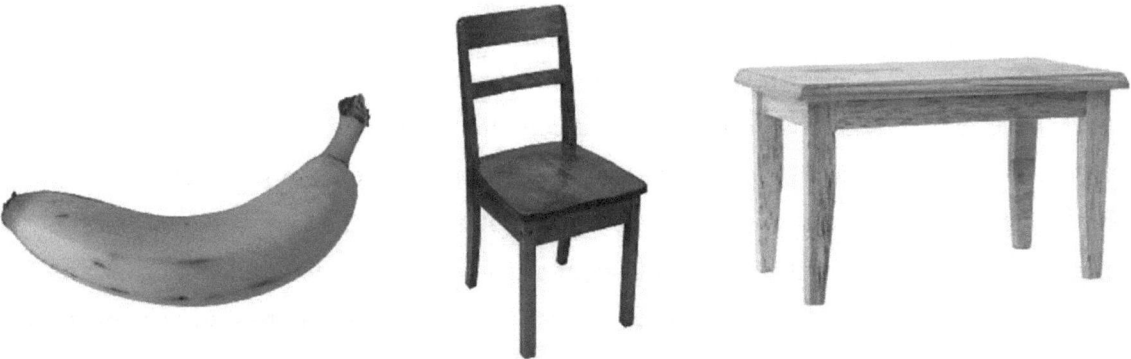

Figure 5.2 Example of an "odd one out" task with a target (banana) that is not semantically related

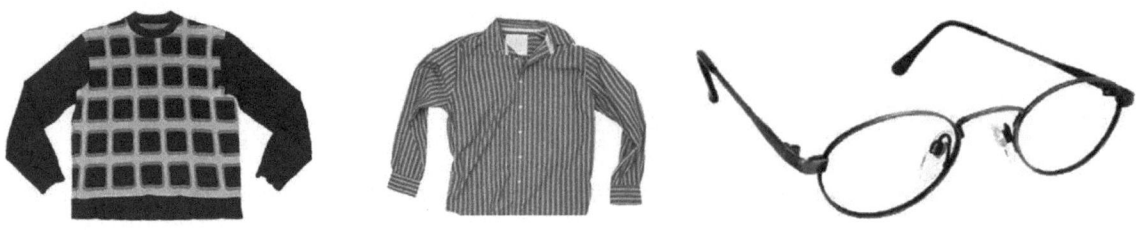

Figure 5.3 Example of an "odd one out" task whereby the target (glasses) that is semantically related to non-target stimuli

In "complete the category" tasks, clients are required to identify from a choice of two pictures which is semantically related to two or more target pictures. Although relying on similar skills to the odd one out task, I have found clients to find this more challenging. Two pictures which belong to the same category are placed in a horizontal row in front of the client. A small space should be left and then two additional pictures presented vertically to the right of the initial two pictures (see Figure 5.4). The SaLT should demonstrate that one of the pictures on the right is connected with the original two whilst one is not connected. This can be done by moving the incorrect option to the target items and saying "no," emphasising with facial expression and gesture that this does not connect and then taking the correct option and placing this with the others. Again, this task can be done non-verbally or verbally. If done verbally, there is no need to over-complicate the instructions and I usually keep to simple words and phrases such as "This here? No," "This here? Yes," "together," "all food," and "all eating." Complexity can again be increased by providing options that are more closely semantically related.

Use of apps

Tactus Therapy Solutions Ltd (2022b) makes a range of language apps for people with aphasia. Within their selection of apps is one called "Category Therapy" which contains non-verbal

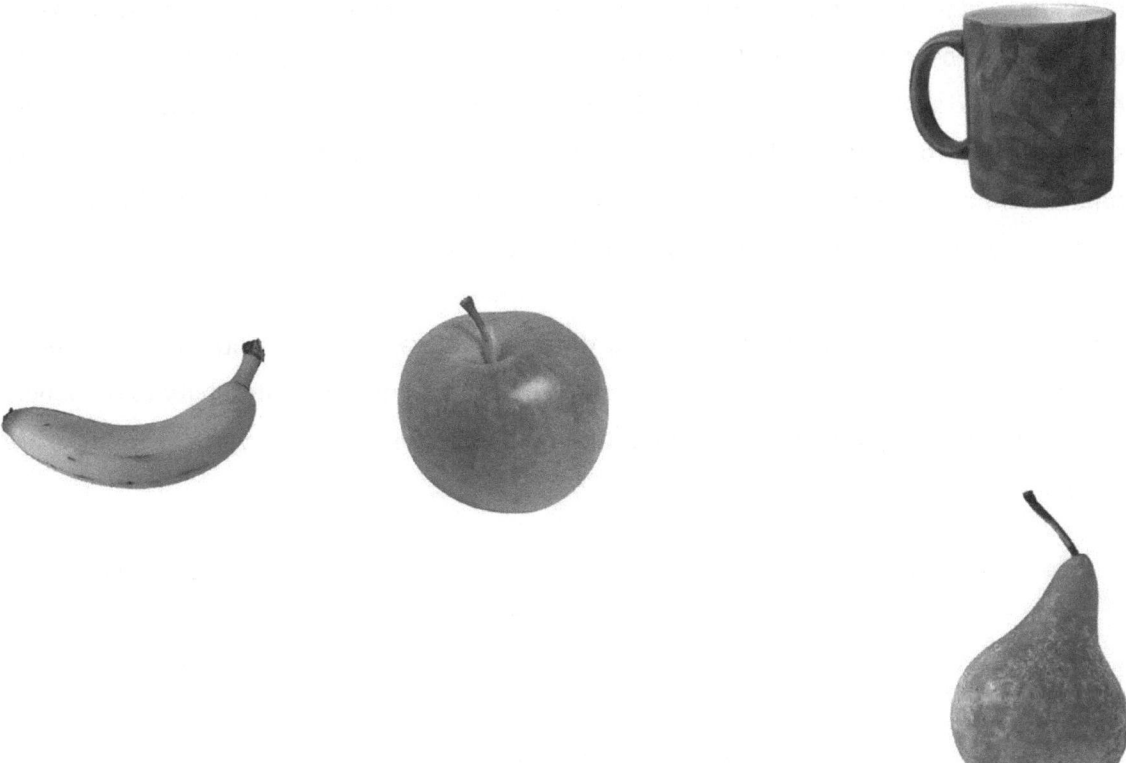

Figure 5.4 Example of a "complete the category" task

semantic tasks, some of which may be useful for PwGA such as Mr B. There are four tasks within the Category Therapy app and the difficulty level can be set as easy, medium, or hard and the number of choices changed to between two and six depending on the task. Further personalisation can occur by using pictures only, written words only, or both written words and pictures as stimuli. When using these apps with PwGA I typically use the picture only version of the task to remove any linguistic demands. Categories used within the tasks can be selected and deselected to ensure all items are relevant and familiar to the individual. It should be noted that the app contains items more culturally relevant to North America and these might need to be deselected if using with PwGA in other parts of the world.

The Cuespeak app (Cuespeak Ltd, 2022) contains non-verbal semantic association tasks with functional stimuli that are extremely useful when working on semantics with clients that have some residual semantic abilities such as matching a verb to an event picture.

Developing comprehension and use of gestures

One of Mr B's goals is to be able to understand and produce a set of gestures. To correctly interpret an iconic gesture, it is necessary to understand the use of the item. Gesture training is therefore about understanding object use and being able to recognise the hand shapes and movements that represent the way in which the object is used. It is important to acknowledge the complexity that exists in this requirement and the underlying skills that need to be established. VAT (Helm-Estabrooks et al., 1982) as outlined in Chapter 4 provides a systematic framework for training underlying semantic and conceptual skills relevant to gesture. Whilst the specific gestures trained in VAT are not particularly functional or relevant to everyday contexts, it is possible to select personally relevant gestures for a specific client and still follow the steps of VAT.

Gesture can also be trained without using VAT and this was the case with Mr B. Instead, a hierarchically ordered set of tasks was used aimed first at improving his ability to recognise actions, then linking actions to objects before finally linking actions to verbs. The tasks are as follows:

- Match a real-life action of the SaLT using an object (such as the SaLT using a comb on their hair) to a physical object (comb) from an array
- Match a real-life action of the SaLT using an object (such as the aforementioned comb) to a picture of an object from an array
- Match an iconic gesture performed by the SaLT to an object/picture
- Match an iconic gesture performed by the SaLT to a verb picture

The number of choices within an array can be gradually increased from two to five or more as performance improves.

In terms of training gesture production, Mr B was initially trained using physical objects. For example, he practiced holding an empty cup and completing the action of drinking, placing a pillow to one side of his head and closing his eyes to indicate sleeping, and so forth. Then over time the physical objects were removed, and Mr B was taught to complete the actions without using the physical objects. He was however initially taught to do this in response to being shown the object. Once doing so accurately, he learnt to produce the action in response to a picture, rather than the physical object. During the therapy process cues may be provided to support clients to complete the relevant gesture such as the following:

- Providing the object
- Physically moulding the client's upper limb/hands/fingers into the correct initial shape or position
- Providing the initial movement and allowing the client to complete the movement
- Demonstrating the gesture and allowing the client to copy the gesture. A point of note relevant to clients with hemiparesis or severe cognitive impairments is to ensure demonstrations involve use of the same side of upper limb(s) the client will use and are shown from the client's position. Seemingly minor differences in the therapist's position place an additional demand on the client (e.g. in having to mirror the SaLT) and increase task difficulty.

Advancing yes/no responses

In the previous case study with Mrs M, yes/no responses were primarily trained through matching tasks and the concept same/different. With Mr B, as there were some functional comprehension and basic semantic skills at baseline, the focus of yes/no training was on understanding these concepts in the context of correct/incorrect using semantic verification tasks. These included Mr B being required to indicate "yes" or "no" as to whether two pictures are connected (semantically) or whether a gesture produced by the SaLT is correct for the target picture or not.

A Yes/No chart can be used in a similar way to the previous case study with Mrs M. However, in clients at Mr B's level with some functional communication skills, I also encourage gestural yes/no responses such as giving a thumbs up/or down and head nodding or shaking especially when there is a therapy goal around gesture. Feedback and correction of errors is essential in yes/no tasks to limit confusion of the already semantically related concepts. Cues in the form of demonstration and physical assistance such as hand moulding for thumbs up/down or placing a hand gently behind the client's head and initiating the initial head movement for yes/no can be provided. It must be said that training clients to use thumbs up/down or head gestures for yes/no can be challenging, especially if limb apraxia is an issue. Training verbal yes/no responses is even more taxing because of the severity of clients' expressive aphasia. Frequently, a Yes/No chart is a more viable option in this population.

Improving auditory single word comprehension

Another of Mr B's goals is to provide a yes/no response to an auditory question about his day during supported conversations. Mr B must understand the question in order to provide an accurate yes/no response and there is consequently a need to work on auditory comprehension. The first step was to agree relevant vocabulary to target. In Mr B's case 12 concrete words were agreed and included some names of carers and other residents in the care home, activities, places, and meals. From this core set three or four words were treated per session. In clients with significant semantic deficits I endeavour to initially select three or four words from the set that are as distinct phonologically and as semantically unrelated as possible. Over time, semantically related or phonologically similar words from the set may be targeted within the same session. To personalise treatment further, photos of the client's own items can be taken and used (if consent is provided). Consistent with the traditional way single words are tested and treated in SLT auditory word-to-picture matching tasks were used to target comprehension of the relevant words. However, an errorless learning approach was used. This is described in the following section.

Errorless learning

Errorless learning involves teaching a client a skill by providing maximal support so that they avoid making errors. The approach is used extensively within cognitive rehabilitation particularly in the field of dementia but has been applied to aphasia and in particular naming therapy (Fillingham, Hodgson, Sage, & Lambon Ralph, 2003; Conroy, Sage, & Lambon Ralph, 2009). Traditionally in naming therapy, clients are shown a picture and asked to name it. Only if the client is unsuccessful are they given cues and usually cues are given hierarchically. For example, the client might be given the semantic category and then asked to re-attempt naming the picture. If unsuccessful they may be given a further cue such as initial phoneme, and if still unsuccessful a further cue and so on until the client may eventually have to be provided with the target. This type of approach is referred to as an "errorful approach" or "retrieval practice." In contrast, errorless learning involves the client being shown a picture and immediately given its name by the SaLT. After the SaLT has named the item, the client is asked to repeat the name. It is thought that errorful approaches can reinforce errors. However, evidence of this in naming therapy is equivocal. Conroy et al. (2009) found no significant difference in the effectiveness of errorless and errorful approaches for naming treatment (i.e. the approaches were as effective as each other). Whilst studies of errorless learning in aphasia have not included PwGA for the obvious reason that they have insufficient spoken output to participate in the naming therapy, I do use the approach regularly in impairment-based tasks. I have found it reduces frustration and struggle and gives clients a sense of satisfaction because they can complete the task accurately and experience success. Many PwGA rarely experience success in therapy, and this risks them becoming despondent, frustrated, and demotivated with SLT. Errorless learning can reduce this risk to a degree.

The following example explains how errorless learning was used to train Mr B in auditory comprehension. One of Mr B's target words was "door" (because he frequently attempts to ask carers for his door to be opened or closed). In the session I would present a picture of a door whilst simultaneously saying the word "door" three times. Mr B would then be asked to "point to the door." Given that he would have just been told three times that the picture was "door" and there was only one picture to choose from, he would consistently respond correctly in keeping with the rationale behind errorless learning. Should a client not respond correctly the process would be repeated until they provide a correct response. Mr B was then presented two additional pictures and words in the same way. Having presented the targets individually using errorless learning, the next step was to present all three pictures simultaneously and remind him of each word. The three pictures were placed on the table in a horizontal row in front of Mr B and each picture was named three times whilst pointing to each picture. Mr B was then asked to point to one of the three items in a random order. At this stage, because there was a choice (in the form of three pictures to select from), errors did occur but were infrequent due to the level of priming provided. When errors occurred, Mr B was shown the correct picture, provided with the verbal label three times, and given another opportunity to select the correct picture. Using this method, many PwGA can learn a small list of functional words.

Advancing auditory comprehension

To advance auditory comprehension skills it is possible to continue with auditory word to picture matching tasks but increase the number of items the client must select from. Another option is to continue with a small selection of three pictures but extend the language within the instruction. For example, rather than saying "point to the door," I may use a Wh-question such as "Where is the door?" I may also add empty language such as "Can you show me where the door is?" or provide a descriptive cue such as "Which one do we open?" The increase in complexity of these step-ups is important for generalisation to function. Too often we target only single words (e.g. the word "drink") in therapy but in functional contexts, the client is being asked full questions such as "What would you like to drink?" In some cases I may emphasise the key word within the phrase ("Where is the picture of the **door**?"). However, over time I try to say the phrases as naturally as possible as a bridge to functional contexts where clients do not necessarily have all communication partners using such strategies. Through use of this approach, I have frequently seen generalisation occur whereby clients can understand their target words in a range of functional contexts.

Other ways of building auditory comprehension in a client of Mr B's level is a variation of the category sorting tasks described earlier. The client is presented with two pictures that represent two different categories such as food (represented by a picture of a meal familiar to the client) and drink (represented by a picture of a drink familiar to the client). Different examples belonging to either category are verbally named by the SaLT (e.g. "milk," "beer," "sandwich") and the client asked to point to the picture representing the category the word belongs to. More than two categories can be used and if preferred written category names provided rather than pictures. This task can be a useful bridge within comprehension intervention in that it provides the client with the opportunity to identify the group a word belongs to without necessarily having to know its exact meaning. Within the collection of tasks in the Tactus Therapy Solutions Ltd (2022b) Category Therapy app is a task called "Find" which is a slightly more advanced variation of this task in which the client is required to listen to the auditorily presented category "food" and find the corresponding item from an array of pictures or written words the one that belongs to this category.

Another app that is useful for developing single word comprehension is Comprehension Therapy found within the Language Therapy app by Tactus Therapy Solutions Ltd (2022a). This requires clients to listen to single words and match them to a picture or written word from a choice of between two and six.

Functional practice and promoting generalisation

Functional practice with yes/no chart

To develop use of the Yes/No chart functionally I often use information gained from the communication history form to engage clients in a supported conversation about their family, hobbies, and preferences, encouraging them to point to a "yes" or "no" in response to questions. An alternative way is to have symbols or written words to represent "yes" and "no" as two separate piles and for clients to place pictorial options of different items (such as foods, drinks, activities) onto each pile according to whether they like or dislike them. To ensure clients maintain turn-taking skills and understand the two-way element of interaction and conversation, I often take my own turns within this task also. When dong so I use gesture, facial expression, spoken key words, and a Yes/No chart to illustrate my preferences thus providing clients with functional demonstration of how they can use non-verbal communication.

Board games

Clients at Mr B's level may be more able to actively participate in basic games than clients such as Mrs M. This can be an engaging way for families to be able to involve their loved one in a meaningful activity. I often demonstrate and support families to engage clients in games such as Snap using a full set of cards, Connect 4, snakes and ladders, or picture lotto and memory games. During these tasks I advise that clients should be encouraged to identify when it is their turn, follow the rules using support and cues, engage in automatic speech such as counting the number of places to move in snakes and ladders, and recognise when someone has won. Clients can also be encouraged to non-verbally congratulate the winner, for example with a high five or thumbs up.

Communication charts or communication books

Communication charts typically contain relevant words, pictures, numbers, alphabet letters, or common phrases to enable people with severe forms of aphasia to make basic requests. These are often generic, containing items deemed relevant to most typical adults. Some are produced by charities such as the Stroke Association. The advantage of these charts is that they are quick and easy for SaLTs to access. Making an individualised chart for a client can be extremely time consuming in a clinical setting and indeed the content required for many clients is similar. However, the issue is that many generic charts have a significant number of pictures on a page and can therefore be very difficult for PwGA to navigate and use effectively. I have found communication charts for PwGA to work best if they contain six or fewer pictures per page. When developing communication charts, additional attention may have to be paid to the size of pictures and layout (such as how much space to leave between pictures) as well as how many semantically similar items are presented on the same page.

In global aphasia a significant amount of training may be needed for clients to use communication charts appropriately within the context required. Many of the interventions discussed thus far may need to be delivered before a communication chart can be introduced such as intervention for visually scanning and shifting gaze, selective attention, and non-verbal semantics.

Once clients can recognise and understand pictures on their communication chart, they must then connect the picture with a functional situation or problem and initiate pointing to the correct picture when they find themselves in that particular situation. One way I have seen clinicians attempt to train clients in this is to provide verbal scenarios to clients such as "Which one would you point to if you are hungry?" or ""Which one would you point to if you are in pain?" I have found this to be a suitable task for clients with relatively spared comprehension abilities. However, this may be too complex for PwGA, not only because of language demands but also due to the hypothetical and abstract nature of the request. I have found many clients instead benefit from seeing the chart used repeatedly in specific contexts. So, for example, every time a nurse comes to give them their medication the nurse might point to the picture of tablets and ask the client to also do so (copy) before giving them their tablet. Or every time the client is given something to drink on the ward the same might have to be done. This develops a link between the picture and the situation as well as development of communicative intent and cause and effect. The client learns to link pointing to a particular picture with a specific situation. Of course, the success of this very much depends on implementation of an MDT approach which requires training and commitment of all involved.

In some cases, clients may reach a point when they are ready to learn the names of items on the chart. In such cases the communication partner should be encouraged to simultaneously name the picture whilst pointing during functional contexts. Another option suitable for developing comprehension of auditory words relevant to a communication chart is to use simple high tech AAC devices such as the GoTalk communication device series (Attainment Company Inc, n.d.). These enable a personalised set of pictures or symbols to be made as an overlay. Depending on the specific GoTalk device used, overlays can accommodate from one to 32 or more pictures and symbols. Each picture/symbol corresponds with one button on the GoTalk device and a word or phrase can be recorded by the SaLT, a relative, or another person to correspond with each picture or symbol. This means that each time a client presses a button on their GoTalk communication chart they hear the recorded word/ phrase and therefore have the opportunity to link the picture or symbol with an auditory word and learn this vocabulary.

Whilst communication charts are often a one-page resource, communication books tend to consist of many pages of pictures. These pictures may relate to basic needs but often they contain personalised information about the client and are intended to be used as an aid for participation in conversations rather than making requests. Typically, they contain personal photos rather than generic pictures or symbols and include information about a client's life history, occupation, family, hobbies and interests, and likes and dislikes. It is important where possible to liaise with family and/or the client as to what they would or would not like included in their communication book. A common issue found clinically is that after spending many hours developing a personalised book for a client, SaLTs find it is rarely used. Often this is because family/carers do not know how to use communication books with the client or the client has not been provided with intervention targeted at its use. Family and carers often require demonstration and training on how to use the communication book functionally. Joint sessions are extremely beneficial as are short training videos of the client and SaLT participating in a supported conversation using the communication book alongside explanations and additional suggestions.

A contents page at the beginning of a communication book can be useful for helping the client and others locate pages relevant to a specific topic. The contents page may contain written words, images, or symbols. Common topics might be family, friends, meals, activities, memorable events, past holidays, music, television, and weather. Functional practice with the book might involve the client finding a specific topic on the contents list and then finding the relevant page. An issue I find with communication books is that whilst they aim to promote conversation, frequently they are used as more of a question-and-answer type "test" in which the communication partner drives the conversation, asks all the questions, and at times asks "test questions" (questions which they may actually know the answer to). It is beneficial to promote two-way conversation in as realistic a way as possible through encouraging the client to both answer questions and initiate or lead communication. One way to do this is to give the client time to scan pages and encourage them to point to a picture of interest to lead the conversation. It is helpful to avoid automatically asking questions should a client point to something of interest. Commenting can be just as effective. It may be a comment such as "that looks like a great holiday" is sufficient to enable a client to give a nod in response where a question such as "where were you?" is too challenging. Most of the interactions PwGA have involve either being asked "test questions" or being asked questions about their wants and needs. Giving comments during interaction tasks is a way to demonstrate that communication can be a way of engaging and sharing based on genuine interest and does not have to follow a question-and-answer format.

A typical session using Mr B's communication book involved being asked what he had done that day and being supported to respond by pointing to relevant pictures in his book and using gestures. After this, Mr B would be asked to select a topic from the contents page of the communication book and find this page. He would then be supported to engage in conversation about the topic not only by answering questions posed to him using pointing and gesture but also asking questions back. Mr B's communication book contained a question page with three simple questions, including "and you?" which was written alongside an image of a finger pointing and a question mark symbol. During the supported conversation, after providing an answer, Mr B was taught to go to the question page and point to the symbol for "and you?" Over time he learnt to ask "and you?" in this way in a range of situations and communication contexts.

Talking photo albums can be used as communication books. These enable a message to be recorded to correspond with each photograph. The messages can be recorded by relatives and provide contextual information to aid facilitation of conversations. Recordings also enable clients to use the albums independently. They can turn pages, press the button to listen to recordings, and hear meaningful personally relevant information.

It is always necessary to see personalised communication charts and books as evolving tools that should be developed and modified over time as clients' preferences, interests, and abilities change. This also makes the book interesting and constantly relevant to the client. A common reason provided by family and carers as to why communication books are not used is that they are out of date. Ideally, family and carers should be guided on how to update the book themselves when needed.

Measuring gains

Mr B achieved all treatment goals after 14 weeks of intervention provided once weekly alongside support and practice with carers. Aside from reviewing achievement of goals, outcomes were measured using the ASHA-FACS (Frattali et al., 1995) rated by his carers and informal functional assessment. Mr B's baseline ability to make a choice, recognise and communicate a mistake, use a Yes/No chart, and gesture within the functional activity of completing a jigsaw puzzle was compared with his ability after intervention. The ASHA-FACS highlighted improvement in social communication, communication of basic needs, and reading, writing, and number concepts. Substantial improvements were also noted in communication partner burden and appropriateness of communication.

Case study 3: Mr P

As outlined in Chapters 1 and 3, Mr P has global aphasia but has retained some single word and functional comprehension abilities. Mr P can repeat words and produce automatic speech. He also has sufficient semantic abilities at baseline to use a communication chart and gesture somewhat successfully. He is however less able to use writing or drawing functionally. It is clients at Mr P's level who may benefit from multimodal approaches (approaches which require use of a range of communication modalities) such as total communication or PACE (Davis & Wilcox, 1981, 1985).

Mr P's goals were to be able to do the following:

- Understand written key words and phrases in his personalised communication book
- Use total communication to engage in conversations with his wife
- Verbally produce targeted single words and set phrases in appropriate contexts

Approaches and tasks that can be used to address these goals are described next.

Promoting spoken output

Functional word lists

A target set of words or short phrases were identified through conversations with family and understanding of Mr P's daily routine and conversation/communication contexts. Mr P's target words and phrases included the following:

- Living room
- Sarah (his daughter)
- Fine, thank you
- And you?

Initially, the items were practiced through a combination of errorless learning and repetition. Then phrase and question cues that had been identified through discussion with Mr P's wife were presented verbally and Mr P was taught to produce the target word in response to the cue. For example, the SaLT would say "You like to watch telly in the. . . ." and Mr P was expected to respond with "living room."

For the more concrete words within the client's target list, images can be used. In the case of Mr P, a photograph of his daughter Sarah and his own living room were used. It is useful to include images where possible to ensure clients link the words or phrases to meaning rather than repeat them or complete phrases in an automatic or parrot-like fashion without understanding what they represent.

Naming

Errorless learning (see Case Study 2, Mr B) is also an effective way of improving naming in PwGA. Sometimes I have combined providing the client with the verbal name three times (consistent with the process of errorless learning) with semantic information. Semantic feature analysis (Boyle, 2010) is a commonly used naming treatment in aphasia. Clients are asked to generate the semantic features of a target concept (usually presented as a picture), for example its category, what it is used for, and where it is located. It is thought that doing this results in strong activation of the target word and increases the likelihood that the individual will be able to name the item. In the context of global aphasia, it is rare a client can generate the semantic information themselves. However, being provided with semantic information is likely to enhance activation in a similar way to if the client generated the information themselves. Providing semantic characteristics verbally alongside images (e.g. providing images of other items in the category or an image of the place in which the item is usually located) is a helpful strategy. The Naming Therapy tasks within Language Therapy (Tactus Therapy Solutions Ltd, 2022a) include a task called "Naming Practice" which enables clients to be provided with a variety of cues to name a target picture. Personally relevant photos can be uploaded and personalised cues also recorded by the therapist.

Script training

Script training is a treatment approach that focuses on improving communication in everyday activities by having the client learn a script that can be used in a specific communication context (Kaye & Cherney, 2016; Hubbard, Nelson, & Richardson, 2020). For Mr P, two simple scripts were produced in collaboration with his wife. These were relevant to placing an order at his favourite restaurant and speaking to his former colleague on a video call. The training typically involves the repeated practice of words and phrases within the script first through repetition, then in unison with the SaLT, and then spontaneously with cues, before finally producing from memory and practicing in the real-life functional context. An example of a script completed with Mr P follows:

Colleague: Hi.

Mr P: Hi, how are you?

Colleague: I'm well, thanks, and you?

Mr P: Fine, thanks. How is work?

Colleague: It's very busy but going well.

Mr P: Busy is good.

Over time, scripts can be extended or clients can learn to generalise to slightly different situations or be provided with a response that is not identical to what they have rehearsed (Goldberg, Haley, & Jacks, 2012).

Single modality non-verbal communication

Although Mr P's goal is to use total communication, it is often helpful to deliver therapy targeting one specific modality at a time first. Therapy for gesture has been discussed in the previous section when describing intervention for Mr B (Case Study 2). This section will focus on therapy for drawing and writing.

Drawing

To use drawing functionally requires independently bringing to mind the visual representation of an idea/concept and translating this into a drawing. It is a relatively complex skill for PwGA because as has been discussed throughout this book there are often semantic issues that negatively impact the ability to accurately access the visual representation of the idea/concept in the first place. Drawing intervention therefore often needs to start with tasks that practice the ability to think of a concept and translate this into a drawing. A task I use frequently is drawing items in a category (such as fruits, vegetables, clothes). If a client struggles with such a task, it is more likely that drawing will not be a viable option functionally. However, if some potential is demonstrated, then intervention would next focus on improving the recognisability of these drawings. Usually, I do this through providing feedback on the client's drawings and suggesting ways items could be more clearly represented. This may involve me re-drawing the item and explicitly highlighting how my version differs to theirs. The client is then encouraged to copy my drawing two or three times. These practiced items are then removed from sight and the client is asked to draw the item again with the aim that there is some incorporation of the suggestions of improvement. When clients need support in drawing therapy, copying and/or tracing pictures are useful step-downs.

Drawing therapy programmes do exist such as that described by Sacchett, Byng, Marshall, and Pound (1999) and the Communicative Drawing Programme designed by

Helm-Estabrooks, Albert, and Nicholas (2014). Both were designed with PwSA in mind and involve hierarchical drawing tasks that would also be suitable for use with PwGA. Sacchett et al. (1999) suggest a range of tasks to target generative drawing such as a client drawing an item to complete a category, drawing items found in a specific location, or drawing items used for a specific task. A task I often use from the Communicative Drawing Programme (Helm-Estabrooks et al., 2014) is one in which the client must complete a drawing that has missing elements or features.

Making drawing functional

As clients become more proficient at drawing, intervention should focus on functional practice. This might involve building drawing tasks into conversation. For example, by engaging in a supported conversation about a specific topic in which both the client and the SaLT use drawing to communicate. It is important that clients see non-verbal communication being used naturally and effectively and that we as SaLTs do all we can to reduce any stigma that might be attached to using non-verbal communication. Using the modalities we are expecting clients to use is essential. Topic ideas to promote functional drawing include food preferences and items found in a wardrobe or refrigerator.

In clients on the border of severe and global aphasia with relatively strong comprehension and cognitive abilities, functional practice may also explore ways that more complex concepts can be depicted through drawing. For example, in the Sacchett et al. (1999) programme there are suggestions on training clients to depict movement, change in ownership, time, directions, and actions in pictures.

Writing

Where clients have retained some ability to spell – as demonstrated through making close approximations at spelling target words when writing, using an alphabet board, or typing/ texting – writing tasks should be attempted in therapy. However, this is a relatively rare occurrence.

Consistent with other tasks described thus far, writing therapy should focus on a target list of functional words relevant to that individual client. Tracing over words or going over dotted words (such as in handwriting books) are useful first steps, followed by copying and writing to dictation. Tasks requiring missing letters to be completed and anagram tasks in which clients must unscramble words are also useful. Throughout these tasks, images should be linked to the words being practiced to ensure the written words are linked to meaning. The Language Therapy (Tactus Therapy Solutions Ltd, 2022a) includes Writing Therapy tasks such as fill in the blank and anagrams. The SaLT can select from a vast list of specific words to be targeted in therapy so that these are relevant to the individual. Depending on the nature of the word list a further step may be written naming (i.e. writing the name of an image). This can be done through use of the task called "Spell What You See" within the earlier mentioned Writing Therapy app, or writing in response to a specific question. The question can be written or auditorily presented. For example, asking questions such as "What is your daughter's name?" or "Who came to visit yesterday?" and then instructing the client to write down the relevant functional word from their list as answer.

Beeson, Rising, and Volk (2003) describe Copy and Recall Treatment for learning the spellings of a target set of words. The treatment involves copying the target written word three times and receiving feedback on accuracy. The target written word is always linked to a picture and after copying has been completed, the written attempts and target are removed and the client is asked to write the word from memory. Beeson et al. (2003) trialled this technique with eight PwSA and reported positive impairment level outcomes for some. They found that the clients who did not respond well to the treatment had semantic deficits at baseline and difficulties with a written lexical decision task. They go on to suggest that clients with severe semantic deficits or difficulties recognising written non-words may not be candidates for this treatment. I have successfully used Copy and Recall Treatment with clients who are at a relatively high level on the global aphasia spectrum. With additional functional practice of the words in the context of total communication and supported conversation I have seen some generalisation to real-life contexts.

Use of letter tiles or spelling by pointing to an alphabet board can be alternative ways to competing all the previous tasks if a client has challenges using a pen, keyboard, or a tablet. When using an alphabet board to spell full words, WM issues mean clients can lose track of which letters they have pointed to previously. It can be useful to write down clients' selections as they are going along to provide them with real-time visual feedback.

Multimodality non-verbal communication

The requirement to use total communication in real-life contexts, that is combine and switch between the use of speech, pictures, gestures, drawing, and writing often requires targeted training in PwGA. Even if the clients are able to use all the modalities individually and/or have received targeted single modality training in specific areas it cannot be assumed that they can automatically generalise to use a range of modalities at the same time.

Multimodal communication training (MMCT; Purdy & Van Dyke, 2011; Purdy & Wallace, 2016) is one technique that is a helpful bridge towards this. It involves using noun pictures as targets and training clients to communicate the picture using different modalities. Initially, the approach included only the four modalities of speech, use of a picture chart, gesture, and writing but drawing was later included. Thus if the picture is a pair of glasses, as part of the treatment, the client must practice verbally producing "glasses," gesturing glasses, drawing a pair of glasses, and pointing to the picture of glasses on a chart or in a book. The aim is for the client to be able to independently convey a pictured item using different modalities without cueing. Perseveration on a previous modality is a significant issue when I have tried this task with PwGA. Over time success at switching can be achieved but it is rare that clients can use all modalities effectively and rarer still that that the switching would occur without cueing. The studies that have used MMCT with PwSA have found there to be variability in response. Purdy and Wallace (2016) describe a client who made minimal gains after the intervention and suggest this is because of baseline semantic and executive functioning deficits. This supports the notion that SaLTs must carefully consider the pre-requisite skills required to successfully use total communication. Too often multimodality communication approaches are seen as the answer for all PwGA, but in reality there are significant practical issues to consider, and intervention to address pre-requisite semantic and cognitive skills may be required first. In the case of Mr P, he had relatively spared semantic and executive functioning abilities so MMCT was used.

Advancing comprehension beyond single words

Given the severity of impairments in global aphasia, it is rarely appropriate to target sentence level comprehension. However, there are cases when this may be suitable, for example if clients show improvement in comprehension over the course of intervention. Typically I use a functional approach to this and agree a target set of phrases or questions relevant to the client's context and create images that link to these sentences. Then, using an errorless learning approach similar to that described for single words, I support the client to link the auditory phrase/question to the image before later asking them to match an auditory sentence to an image from a choice of two or three. Similarly, if written comprehension is the target, the client is initially presented with the written sentence and the target image and later asked to match a written sentence to an image from a choice. Another task is written phrase completion in which clients must select from a choice of written words the correct one to complete a written phrase. Stimuli can be personalised or reading tasks within the Language Therapy app (Tactus Therapy Solutions Ltd, 2022a) such as written phrase completion can be used.

Functional practice and promoting generalisation

Barrier games such as PACE (Davis & Wilcox, 1981, 1985) detailed in Chapter 4 are highly effective ways of developing use of total communication in a more functional way. In functional contexts the listener does not know the message, and barrier games mimic this in that a client has a picture they have to convey which the listener cannot see. Barrier tasks also enable clients to develop skills in recognising when a modality is not working and trying an alternative approach. They are a useful bridge into practicing total communication within a more conversational context.

In sessions with Mr P, functional use of total communication was practiced through supported conversation in which both he and the SaLT used total communication to express themselves and ask each other questions. Joint sessions with family occurred regularly to ensure consistent use of strategies outside of sessions. Mr P also benefitted from attending group sessions which provided opportunity for functional practice.

Measuring gains

Mr P received intervention twice weekly for eight weeks. He achieved all goals but remained reliant on prompting to use total communication. In particular, he struggled to independently switch to a different modality. In comparison to those with more severe global aphasia, clients at Mr P's level are often able to show gains on formal assessments. Mr P improved on the single word comprehension subtests of the AST (Whurr, 2011), scoring 5/5 on auditory word to object and auditory word to picture matching and 4/5 on written word to picture matching. At baseline the CAT (Swinburn et al., 2004) was attempted but abandoned due to the severity of Mr P's deficits. In such situations it is useful to re-attempt failed assessments after intervention. This can highlight improvements in language, cognitive skills and ability to understand assessment requirements. Indeed, Mr P was able to complete the spoken word and written word comprehension subtests from the CAT after intervention and scored 7/15 and 9/15 respectively. He also made gains on the ASHA-FACS (Frattali et al., 1995) with improvements in the areas of reading and writing and daily planning. In addition, gains in communication partner burden were observed. Anecdotal improvements were also noted by Mr P's family in terms of his spoken output. For example, he reportedly produced recognisable words and phrases spontaneously more frequently.

Group therapy

There is little to no literature on the use of group therapy in global aphasia. In my experience it is best used with clients with relatively good sustained and selective attention, WM, and semantic skills because the cognitive demands required to engage in a group setting are high. Often, groups for PwGA focus on total communication. For example, Lawson and Fawcus (1999) described the use of a total communication group with a client with global aphasia (TS). Tasks included signing, PACE (Davis & Wilcox, 1981, 1985), miming, drawing, reading, and writing. Cognitive skills such as turn-taking, self-monitoring, and evaluating the performance of self and others were also indirectly trained. After treatment, TS is reported to have improved in his ability to use gesture, drawing, and mime in real-life situations but these improvements were not objectively measured. MMCT (Purdy & Van Dyke, 2011; Purdy & Wallace, 2016) has not been investigated as a group intervention, but I have adapted it for use in groups by providing a target and asking each client in turn to communicate the picture in one modality that is different to the previous client. This is a useful stepping-stone to the client having to communicate the item using more than one modality themselves but also encourages turn-taking and recall of what modalities have already been used. Often, I complete MMCT as a warm up task prior to barrier games such as PACE whereby clients are encouraged to use multiple modalities. If conducting groups with more severely impaired clients, I often include non-linguistic group activities such as all contributing to a jigsaw puzzle or a group card or board game to develop turn-taking and cognitive skills such as problem solving. These tasks can also be used to target yes/no whereby clients are encouraged to use their Yes/No charts or non-verbal communication to communicate whether for example two cards match or a jigsaw piece has been placed correctly. Finally, "complete the category" or "odd one out" can be engaging semantic tasks to complete as a group.

Part 2: indirect therapy

Environmental approaches to aphasia have been described by authors such as Lubinski (1981) and Howe, Worrall, and Hickson (2004). The goal is to provide a positive communication environment in which individuals have access to communication opportunities, are valued as meaningful communication partners and where physical barriers to communication are removed. One of the main ways this is manifested is in the provision of communication strategies or communication training to other professionals or family and friends of the client. For a variety of reasons it is often the primary approach used with PwGA. Indirect therapy can often be preferred in the early stages when the client might not be ready for direct intervention due to fatigue, low mood, or medical complications. As discussed, the severity of stroke that induces global aphasia means that often clients are dealing with other stroke related issues, especially in the early stages and direct therapy is not appropriate. However, I would always advocate for PwGA to be offered direct intervention at some point in their journey and for conversation partner intervention to complement this.

Indirect intervention may take the form of written communication strategies provided in medical notes or in a client's room so that family and/or members of an MDT can easily see them. Communication strategies that might be useful for PwGA are listed in Appendix 4. In community or rehabilitation contexts in which SaLTs may have more time available, it can be useful to create a video that carers and family can easily access whereby I demonstrate using the strategies with the individual client. We often take for granted that people can make sense of written strategies and implement without specific guidance. At the very least training or education sessions should be offered to explain and demonstrate these strategies rather than expecting professionals or family to do this with written information alone.

Communication partner training

The environmental approach also includes creating skilled empathetic communication partners through stroke education for relatives, family groups, and staff. Common approaches include Supported Conversations for Adults with Aphasia (SCA; Kagan, 1999), Better Conversations with Aphasia (BCA; Beeke et al., 2013), communication partner training (Blom Johansson, Carlsson, Ostberg, & Sonnander, 2013; Saldert, Backman, & Hartelius, 2013), and Supporting Partners of People with Aphasia in Relationships and Conversation (SPPARC; Lock et al., 2001). Some approaches involve working only with communication partners and others such as BCA and SPPARC involve working with a dyad (both the person with aphasia and their communication partner) but the ultimate aim with all approaches is to improve the skill of the communication partner in using strategies to support conversations. As discussed in Chapter 4, conversations in the true sense of the word are difficult when dealing with people who have limited receptive and expressive abilities and in some cases cognitive impairments too. Authors such as Kagan (1999) suggest conversation partner training may not be suitable for those with very severe impairments. I have adapted the approach to involve training communication partners to improve their interactions (rather than conversations) with PwGA and provide suggestions and strategies for engaging clients in activities. Often, I ask relatives to observe a session (or video) in which I am engaging in an activity with the person with aphasia and then spend time reviewing and discussing strategies I have used to gain active participation and develop basic communication skills. Suggestions include encouraging their loved one with global aphasia to make eye contact, choose an activity, make choices within games (such as what colour counter to have), monitor whose turn it is in a game, answer questions related to the activity such as "Who is winning/losing?" and "Whose turn is it next?". I also encourage inclusion of surprises or mistakes in activities to promote problem solving and reasoning. As described for Mrs M this can be done through breaking game rules, taking a turn in the wrong place, or incorrectly identifying a win. Clients should be encouraged to initiate communicating that there is an error/problem and where appropriate supported to suggest solutions.

In many conversation partner approaches video recording is used. For example, in BCA dyads are encouraged to record themselves engaging in a conversation and sessions involve reviewing these recordings and identifying behaviours and strategies that work well or could be completed differently. In the same way, I have asked dyads to record themselves engaging in an activity such as looking through photos, playing a card or board game, or completing a jigsaw puzzle and then reviewed the recordings and considered strategies that can be used and developed to enhance interaction or communication in this context.

Adapting the environment

Adaptations to the environment can enhance communication for people with language and cognitive difficulties. Environmental factors that have been found to impact successful communication include lighting, acoustic environment, humidity and temperature, setting and furniture placement, and availability of written information or AAC (Stans, Dalemans, de Witte, Smeets, & Beurskens, 2017). Examples of ways that the environment can be adapted for an optimal communication environment for PwGA include ensuring there is a good light source and that the face of the person speaking is clearly visible with no shadows, reducing background noise, and limiting visual distractions. In institutions such as care homes it can be helpful to have carpets, softer furniture, and drapes in larger rooms to absorb sound and reduce reverberation as well as to colour code different areas and label rooms with images to enhance orientation.

Ways to make written information accessible to PwA have been clearly described in the literature. Using simplified language, including clear non-ambiguous images, using font size 14-16 and boldfacing key words are amongst recommendations that have been made (see for example Herbert, Gregory, & Haw, 2019). Given the severity of linguistic impairments in global aphasia the most helpful adaptation to material is the inclusion of images and limiting written language to single words or short phrases with boldfaced key words wherever possible. When considering the use of images, generally pictures and photographs are more meaningful than symbols for this population.

Chapter summary

Using the profiles of three clients with varying severities of global aphasia, this chapter has detailed different intervention tasks that can be used to address non-verbal cognition, language and functional communication at an impairment, functional and social participation level. Examples of resources have been provided and ways of reducing or increasing task complexity suggested. The chapter has emphasised the importance of considering the individual client's cultural background, preferences, and communication contexts when selecting approaches and task items to maximise relevance, promote generalisation, and increase the likelihood of overall positive outcomes.

6

CONSIDERATIONS FOR CLINICAL PRACTICE

Introduction

This final chapter outlines key areas that are important for effective management of PwGA and can influence outcomes.

Multidisciplinary team (MDT) working

SaLTs working with PwGA often work jointly with members of the MDT. Most commonly this is OT but also physiotherapy and psychology. According to a UK survey of clinical practice, capacity and mood assessments are the areas of most collaborative work with other professionals (Adjei, 2015; Adjei-Nicol, 2020). Multidisciplinary working involves drawing on knowledge from another discipline but staying within the boundaries of one's own profession. Interdisciplinary working on the other hand involves working in a more integrated and coordinated way where they may be some blurring of professional boundaries (Choi & Pak, 2006). MDT working may involve SaLTs providing training or joint sessions to model communication strategies and facilitate colleagues to communicate effectively with clients. It may also involve SaLTs modifying information (e.g. simplifying instructions or providing aphasia friendly materials) to enable clients to effectively engage in sessions with other MDT members.

Observation of clients in sessions with other disciplines is another example of multidisciplinary working. It enables information on a client's ability to follow instructions, make choices, recognise objects, and problem solve in more meaningful contexts to be gained. Observation in functional activities such as an OT wash and dress or meal preparation session can be particularly informative. The meaningful contexts of such sessions allow clients to demonstrate areas of strength that would otherwise be missed if only informal

DOI: 10.4324/9781003184522-6

and formal SLT assessments are relied on. OT assessments are often conducted in a room that mimics real life such as a kitchen and involve the use of objects related to the task at hand. Such assessments are also often completed with meaningful intent (e.g. a wash and dress is conducted in the morning when the client needs to get dressed), whereas SLT assessments are often conducted at bedside or in a clinic room using random pictures and objects unrelated to task or setting. As such SLT assessments are inherently more abstract and can lead to clients not fully demonstrating their potential.

Observation of physiotherapy sessions can be extremely useful for ascertaining a client's ability to follow instructions in context, such as whole-body commands. I also often use joint physiotherapy sessions to assess clients' abilities to follow instructions or communicate when distracted. An example might be asking a client to complete a non-verbal task such as picture sorting or "odd one out" whilst the physiotherapist is completing passive movements. This can be used to provide functional examples of how cognitive demands may change the client's performance. In more profoundly impaired clients, determining whether positional changes (such as sitting on the edge of a bed or sitting in a chair) impacts alertness, awareness, or general communicative performance can also be useful to assess in joint sessions with physiotherapy.

An example of interdisciplinary working is joint goal setting. In the context of working with PwGA joint goals often centre on the impact of cognition. Cognition has been a key theme throughout this book. Chapter 1 detailed that many PwGA have severe cognitive deficits alongside their language impairments. Chapter 3 included details on how to assess cognition in aphasia and many interventions for global aphasia described in Chapters 4 and 5 target cognition alongside or instead of language. Yet cognition has historically had little focus in SLT training curricula and many SaLTs do not feel confident in working in this area. OT and neuropsychology have more in-depth knowledge of cognition than SLT and are often the lead providers of cognitive assessment and intervention in neuro-rehabilitation settings. However, professionals in those fields may lack knowledge and skill in working with people with the severe linguistic deficits found in global aphasia, and without input from SLT may not fully appreciate how cognition may be impacting a client's communication. There is a need for interdisciplinary working in this context to bring the different areas of expertise together and gain a more comprehensive understanding of the client. This then allows for holistic goals to be set.

Joint goal setting can positively influence functional outcomes and promote generalisation. It is important though that members of the MDT discuss and agree how each discipline will contribute to shared goals to avoid confusion and duplication. A common joint goal set with OT reported by SaLTs is for the client to be able to make choices in daily activities such as meal times, choosing what to wear, and choosing an activity to engage in (Adjei, 2015, Adjei-Nicol, 2020). With more advanced clients it may be possible to work on more complex goals such as the client following a set of instructions related to a functional task (e.g. a recipe) with the SaLT providing strategies and visual resources to help the client with sequencing and understanding of instructions. Another area of joint work with OT may be in supporting clients' functional communication skills (such as initiation, turn-taking, or use of non-verbal communication) in leisure activities or within community settings.

Neuropsychology assessment typically involves the completion of a battery of cognitive assessments alongside observation of behaviour and evaluation of client self-reports. PwGA often struggle to complete the battery of assessments due to their linguistic deficits and because the assessments are standardised, modifications are not possible. Non-verbal tests may be possible for some PwGA to complete but equally problematic for others due to task instructions and demands. As has been discussed throughout this book, cognitive deficits in joint attention, semantics, and visual perception are common in global aphasia and may preclude any form of formal assessment being completed. SaLTs can however aid clients' participation in psychology sessions by providing strategies to facilitate the client communicating and self-rating their mood or emotions (e.g. visual scales, pictures, or symbols). On some occasions direct intervention to enable this may be required. For example, semantic tasks such as categorisation completed in SLT may be extended to more abstract categories such as emotions. A non-verbal task I have used is for clients to sort picture scenarios into categories based on how the people in the photograph are likely to be feeling. For example, the client may be shown photos of a person getting married, a person attending a funeral, a couple having an argument, and a person lying in a hospital bed and asked to infer the likely emotion being felt by placing each photo under the relevant pile based on a choice of happy, sad, or angry. These emotions might be represented as symbols or emojis. Another task involves clients matching a symbol or emoji of an emotion either to a photograph/scenario of a person expressing the same emotion. This task can help train clients to recognise symbolic representations of feelings which some find difficult. The Inference Pics app (Aptus Speech Therapy, 2020) has hundreds of photo scenarios useful for creating such tasks. The description task within the Advanced Naming Therapy app (Tactus Therapy Solutions Ltd, 2022c) also contains photo scenarios that can be used. As accuracy in the previous tasks improves, clients may then be able to select an emotion to represent their own feelings when given a pictorial scenario. For example, a photo of the nursing home they will be discharged to may be presented and the client asked to select from an array of emotions how they feel about this. Using numerical scales to determine the strength of feeling about an issue is usually not possible with PwGA but use of a modified visual scale with different colours and emojis to differentiate strength of feeling might be possible with the more able clients. An example is provided in Appendix 3.

Neurologic Music Therapy (NMT) is a relatively new field within neurorehabilitation. It involves the use of clinical and evidence-based music interventions to accomplish individualised goals and can positively influence mood, cognition, language, social skills, and physical, communicative, and social needs (Magee, 2019). Although not routinely part of rehabilitation teams, when I have had access to music therapists, I have found joint working on areas such as initiation, turn-taking, and attention through for example the client listening to and copying rhythmic patterns useful. I have also used same/different tasks using musical stimuli to train clients in the concepts of "yes" and "no." MIT (Albert, Sparks, & Helm, 1973) discussed in Chapter 4 is an obvious approach that lends itself to joint working with music therapy. For clients who have an overlay of severe apraxia of speech I have also worked jointly with music therapists to facilitate spontaneous spoken output through singing or completing the lines of a familiar song using a technique called Musical Speech Stimulation (Thaut, 2005). For those with difficulties initiating or producing voice, techniques using sound vocalisations and wind instruments can be used to aid articulatory control and breath support. A music therapy approach called Symbolic Communication Training Through Music (SYCOM; Thaut, 2016) can be particularly helpful for use with PwGA. The intervention was designed specifically for people with little to no expressive language and/or cognitive impairments and involves a systematic protocol using music patterns and improvisation exercises to develop skills in turn-taking, gesturing, listening and responding, and initiating and terminating communication. I have found the use of NMT alongside SLT to be beneficial for many PwGA but accessibility is an issue and more research about its benefits for this population is required.

Measuring change

The severity of impairment in global aphasia means that often any improvements after intervention may be relatively small. This is highlighted in the studies described in Chapter 4. It is becoming increasingly important for commissioning and funding reasons to be able to provide evidence of benefit of SLT. Selecting the most appropriate ways to demonstrate change is therefore essential. In global aphasia, SaLTs should ensure that outcomes do not just focus on accuracy and assessment scores but also capture improvements in levels of initiation, speed of response, amount of demonstration required to understand a task, amount of cueing required to respond, and the level of communication burden the communication partner or relative carries. For example, if a client's comprehension of gesture and processing speed improves after intervention, this may lead to a reduction in the amount of demonstration, repetition, or cueing a relative needs to provide before the client can engage in an activity as well as a reduction in the amount of time the relative must wait for a response. These examples equate to an improvement in the efficiency and quality of interactions that reduce the level of burden for the communication partner. There may be positive implications for the relative's mood or quality of life as a result of this which may indirectly impact the client's mood also. This domino effect highlights that relatively small changes can have significant functional implications. Yet often these changes are not captured or articulated by SaLTs and the vital benefits of SLT may go unnoticed.

SaLTs should attempt to use assessments more likely to draw out small subtle changes in this population. Some examples from Chapter 3 include the BNVRT (Butt & Bucks, 2004), the ASHA-FACS (Frattaliet al., 1995) or use of Talking Mats in combination with the COPM (Law et al., 2019) to compare ratings of performance at baseline with those after intervention. The Carers COAST (Long, Hesketh, & Bowen, 2009) is a carer related outcome measure that through a self-rating questionnaire before and after intervention can also be used to demonstrate changes in carer quality of life.

Intervention practices

Timing of intervention

The evidence presented in Chapter 4 suggests that PwGA can make improvements many years after the initial onset of symptoms. Indeed, most intervention studies have involved clients in the chronic stage. The evidence also suggests that the trajectory of recovering in the condition may be longer than for other aphasias, with the most substantial gains often made more than six months after onset (Sarno & Levita, 1981; Smania et al., 2010). Yet clients and relatives are often told that they should expect most gains in the first six months and limited gains thereafter. Many rehabilitation services often provide the most amount of SLT within the first six months post onset and less (if any) in the more chronic stages. Subsequently, PwGA are often not being provided with intervention at the time they will most benefit from it. A further issue is that the severity of stroke or brain injury that induces global aphasia means that it may take clients longer to become medically stable enough to fully engage and benefit from SLT. A final consideration is that if clients retain some insight into their condition, the impact of the profound changes to their communication and life more broadly may impact mood and motivation thus further limiting their ability to participate and make maximal gains from SLT. To reflect current evidence and NHS priorities around person-centred care, models of delivery for PwGA should ideally be as flexible as possible, allowing for intervention at different stages of recovery depending on the individual.

Dose and intensity

"Dose" refers to the overall amount (total number of hours) of intervention provided. "Intensity" refers to the number of hours per a week an intervention is provided. The consensus from existing evidence detailed in Chapter 4 and summarised in the previous section suggests that PwGA may require a larger dose of intervention over a longer period than those with other forms. However, in my recent study (Adjei-Nicol, 2020) participants made functional gains after an average of nine sessions. This finding demonstrates that it is possible for PwGA to improve with standard doses of intervention. Response to intervention is likely dependent on the content and approach used.

The evidence is conflicting when considering whether PwGA benefit from intensive intervention. There is also conflicting evidence about the benefits of intensive intervention in the broader aphasia literature. Bhogal, Teasell, and Speechley (2003) completed a systematic review and found intensive intervention led to more favourable SLT outcomes. On the other hand, Cherney, Patterson, and Raymer (2011) found no clear difference in outcome between high and low intensity delivery in their systematic review. Furthermore, there are studies such as those by Dignam et al. (2015) which have found a distributed (less intensive) delivery to lead to more favourable outcomes than the same intervention delivered intensively. The only study to specifically explore intensity in global aphasia was the study by Denes et al. (1996) detailed in Chapter 4. This study reported an advantage for intensive SLT but had methodological issues and only marginal differences between the intensive and regular intervention groups.

As also discussed in Chapter 4, there is emerging evidence that an Intensive Comprehensive Aphasia Programme (ICAP) can improve outcomes after SLT. Rose et al. (2013) define key elements of ICAPs and explain that they must involve a minimum of three hours treatment daily for at least two weeks. Importantly, a key component of ICAPs is the inclusion of a variety of different treatment approaches such as individual and group therapy as well as tasks targeting impairment, functional activities, and social participation. ICAPs must also include education support for the individual and for families, have a defined start and end date, and involve a set cohort of individuals entering and leaving the programme at the same time. Leff et al. (2021) report large gains in language and functional measures after their ICAP as well as maintenance of these gains at follow up. Other ICAP studies such as Hoover, Caplan, Waters, and Carney (2017) have had similarly positive outcomes. Given these promising findings, some NHS services are beginning to trial and explore this mode of service delivery for aphasia. The problem currently is that we do not know whether PwGA can benefit from ICAPs in the same way as those with other forms of aphasia. PwGA have generally not been included in ICAP studies to date and if they have, due to analysis taking place at the group level, it is not possible to understand the degree to which they have been able to participate or benefit. One probable challenge for PwGA participating in ICAPs is the issue of fatigue. Generally, due to the size of lesions and severity of brain damage that induces global aphasia, clients are more susceptible to fatigue effects. It is likely some will have difficulty tolerating three hours or more a day of intervention. Another issue is the need for intervention in ICAPs to be comprehensive (i.e. use a range of approaches and target multiple different areas). It may be that again due to the degree of impairment this is overwhelming for some PwGA and overloads what is already a suppressed cognitive system. I have known clients to experience such cognitive overload from multiple rehabilitation sessions, leisure activities, and visitors in one day that there is a "shutting down" of the system – a reduction in responses and overall performance. It may be that some PwGA require "readiness" therapy prior to engaging in ICAPs. As research into ICAPs expands the hope is that we gain more understanding of how this model of delivery can be effectively applied to PwGA.

Remote therapy

Teletherapy, sometimes referred to as "telerehabilitation," involves intervention being delivered using digital technology such as video conference calling. Previously this method was often used to deliver services to clients who had difficulty accessing services due to location or mobility. However, teletherapy has become embedded into many clinical settings as a result of the global COVID-19 pandemic which commenced in 2020. Generally, research findings suggest teletherapy is as effective as in-person therapy for aphasia (Cherney & van Vuuren, 2012; Woolf et al., 2016; Cacciante et al., 2021). However, there are little to no examples of successful use with PwGA. One issue is that PwGA rely heavily on non-verbal cues and total communication which can be difficult in video calls. For example, gestures may be difficult to see, or if a client uses writing or drawing, they must be able to navigate using and sharing a whiteboard or holding up their written attempts to the screen.

PwGA may have additional deficits such as hemiparesis, visual neglect, or hemianopia that impact ability to see all parts of the screen or use and navigate the technology. One of the main challenges I have found is the attentional demands required. For example, clients find it difficult to switch attention between the presenter and material shared on the screen or to follow information shared without having a clear view of the presenter. Some clients also get distracted seeing their own faces on the video. Generally, I have found teletherapy possible with this population only if the main focus of the session is to work on verbal (spoken) output and the client has relatively spared cognition. In such cases there has been little to no need to use other forms of communication within the session and the client has the attention and executive function ability to appropriately focus, navigate the technology, and respond to any technical issues that may arise.

Discharging clients

Often, service specifications influence when a client must be discharged. However, ideally the main factor should be whether the client is making gains. One way of measuring this is to ascertain whether the client has achieved goals. However, SaLTs must be cautious with this. If a client has not achieved goals, this does not necessarily mean they are unable to benefit from SLT. More often than not, it means that a component within the intervention process requires adjusting. Perhaps the goal is too challenging and requires stepping down, or the intervention approach used to address the goal could be altered, or the client has had insufficient opportunities for practice outside SLT sessions, or client mood or motivation is an issue that requires exploring with other members of the MDT.

Other times, discharge decisions may be made based on whether improvements have been noted on outcome measures. As detailed earlier in this chapter, careful consideration of the way in which changes are measured is required to ensure that subtle or indirect gains are captured. I have frequently disagreed with claims that clients are "unable to benefit from intervention" or when "the severity of impairments" is used as a rationale for limited intervention or discharge. Whilst some intervention approaches will indeed be impossible for the more profoundly impaired individual, it is extremely rare for there to be no role for SLT. Sometimes the issue is that dose of intervention provided is insufficient. It may also be that SaLTs must explore novel ways of working with the client such as providing "readiness" intervention in pre-requisite cognitive skills relevant to SLT, for example joint attention and non-verbal semantics. All reasonable effort should have been made before discharging clients on the basis of perceived lack of rehabilitation potential.

Discharge can be a difficult time for clients and relatives, as they may feel abandoned and anxious about the future. It is an important time to offer hope despite the chronic nature of the client's condition. I remind relatives that clients may continue to make small gains over many years even without SLT. To offer hope I further emphasise that as research in the field is limited there is still much to understand and discover. New knowledge and insights that may benefit their loved one in the future may yet come.

Working with clients from culturally diverse backgrounds

I have emphasised throughout this book the need to personalise intervention by considering the client's cultural background, beliefs, and communication contexts during the entire therapeutic process. This applies to all clients whether they are from a diverse background or not. Time must be invested in gaining information from family, friends, or other key people relevant to that client (e.g. a religious leader) at the start of the client's journey. Information gained should then be used to inform decisions such as which language sessions intervention will be conducted in, who needs to be involved in SLT, which assessment items may not be familiar to the client and need to be skipped, what alternative label a client may have used for a specific word that we need to be aware of, and much more.

Given the extensive use of pictures in SLT and the importance of developing non-verbal semantic skills in this population, a key factor to consider is the images used as stimuli and whether they depict an item in a way that would be most familiar for the client. For example, if a target word is "slipper" and the picture used in therapy to represent this word is a fluffy slipper often worn indoors this may not evoke meaning for a client from a different background in the same way that say an image of a pair of flip-flops would. It is important to use not just functionally relevant vocabulary but also familiar images and visual representations of items. Similarly, prior to working on non-verbal communication such as eye contact or gestures, family should be consulted about the appropriateness of this, and the SaLT should check that intended actions have the same meaning across cultures.

Interpreters may need to be used in some cases and this can be challenging when working with PwGA, as ideally we require them to not only translate words but also modify or simplify the message and potentially use non-verbal communication alongside. Additional time may be required to educate and prepare interpreters for this but often in busy clinical settings this is not possible.

Finally, there is the need to consider a client's beliefs about illness, the medical field, and the rehabilitation process. Beliefs may link with the client's cultural background and influence opinion on prognosis and the value of SLT. This needs to be carefully considered when providing education about the condition, information on prognosis, or rationale for specific SLT interventions.

Where next in global aphasia?

Use of non-linguistic and non-verbal interventions

Research and clinical experience suggest there is an advantage to conducting interventions focused on cognition rather than language in this population and doing so non-verbally. However, significantly more research is required on this and indeed in global aphasia more broadly. The feasibility of non-linguistic and non-verbal interventions becoming common practice will likely be influenced by historical and institutional practices. Many SaLTs do not feel confident in their knowledge of or skills in working on cognition. There are further issues about SLT training in this area and overlapping roles with other MDT members which require exploring.

Expanding the evidence base

A theme throughout this book has been the lack of research with this population. This is the main contributory factor to the lack of resources available for use with the population and the reduced confidence many SaLTs have in working with this client group. One reason often cited in research studies for excluding PwGA is their limited comprehension abilities or difficulties with consent. A further factor is recruitment. Many intervention studies seek participants who are more than six months post stroke and recruit from stroke groups or SLT services. Yet it is common for PwGA to no longer be receiving intervention six months post onset, either due to service constraints or due to the perception they have not made gains or are unable to benefit from SLT. PwGA have often had severely disabling strokes that mean they need significant amounts of care and may reside in institutions such as nursing homes. They are also frequently unable to attend stroke groups due to mobility and access issues or because the severity of their impairments limits their ability to participate. All of these issues mean that finding PwGA to participate in research is a challenge. Usually, PwGA cannot consent themselves. The Mental Capacity Act (2005) advises that people lacking consent should be given as much help and support as possible to express their own opinion about participating in a study. Where this is not possible, the Act details how a personal consultee can be used. A consultee is an individual prepared to give an opinion as to whether the person lacking capacity to consent would want to take part in the research study. The only condition placed on who a consultee should be is that they are required to know the participant personally (i.e. not in a professional or paid capacity). The client lacking capacity should be supported to give an opinion on who their consultee should be wherever possible. Processes clearly exist to enable PwGA to participate in research but there are limited opportunities. At the point of discharge, it can also be useful to ask next of kin if they are willing to be contacted in the future should a research opportunity for their loved one arise. By keeping informed of current research studies (through engagement with social media, attendance at courses and conferences, and linking in with academic institutions), maintaining skills in appraising the literature, and completing small scale research in the workplace, SaLTs can contribute to the evidence base and support willing clients to participate in research.

Chapter summary

This chapter has highlighted the importance of MDT working and provided suggestions for joint goals and ways of working with OT, physiotherapy, psychology, and music therapy. It has re-iterated the importance of using sensitive outcome measures in the population and discussed when and how discharge might be considered. The chapter has also demonstrated where there are gaps in current knowledge with respect to this population. Specifically, there is limited understanding about optimal dose and intensity, whether ICAPs are effective in global aphasia, and the efficacy of cognitive interventions. Despite the limited literature much can be done clinically and this book provides a wealth of examples to support SaLTs in their everyday practice.

REFERENCES

Adjei, S. (2015, November). Global aphasia: Current perspectives and future directions. *RCSLT Bulletin, 2015*(763), 18-20.

Adjei-Nicol, S. K. (2020). *An investigation into the effect of a novel non-linguistic cognitive intervention on functional communication in global aphasia.* [Doctoral thesis, UCL (University College London)]. UCL Discovery. https://discovery.ucl.ac.uk/id/eprint/10107050/

Agrell, B., & Dehlin, O. (1998). The clock-drawing test. *Age & Ageing, 41*(3), S41-45.

Albert, M., Sparks, R., & Helm, N. (1973). Melodic intonation therapy for aphasia. *Archives of Neurology, 29*, 130-131.

Aptus Speech Therapy Ltd. (2020). *Inference pics* (version 1.4) [Mobile app]. https://www.aptus-slt.com/inference-pics

Atkinson, R., & Shiffrin, R. (1968). Human memory: A proposed system and its control processes. *Psychology of Learning and Motivation, 2*, 89-195.

Attainment Company Inc. (n.d.). *Go talk+ series*. www.attainmentcompany.com/technology/communication-aids

Baddeley, A. (2012). Working memory: Theories, models, and controversies. *Annual Review of Psychology, 63*, 1-29.

Baddeley, A., & Hitch, G. (1974). Working memory. *Psychology of Learning and Motivation, 8*, 47-89.

Basso, A. (2010). "Natural" conversation: A treatment for severe aphasia. *Aphasiology, 24*(4), 466-479.

Beeke, S., Sirman, N., Beckley, F., Maxim, J., Edwards, S., Swinburn, K., & Best, W. (2013). *Better conversations with aphasia: An e-learning resource*. www.ucl.ac.uk/short-courses/search-courses/better-conversations-aphasia-e-learning-resource

Beeson, P. M., Rising, K., & Volk, J. (2003). Writing treatment for severe aphasia: Who benefits? *Journal of Speech, Language, and Hearing Research, 46*(5), 1038-1060.

Beukelman, D., & Mirenda, P. (1998). *Augmentative and alternative communication: Management of severe communication disorders in children and adults* (2nd ed.). Baltimore: P.H. Brookes Publishing.

Bhogal, S. K., Teasell, R., & Speechley, M. (2003). Intensity of aphasia therapy, impact on recovery. *Stroke, 34*(4), 987-993.

Binder, J. R., Desai, R. H., Graves, W. W., & Conant, L. L. (2009). Where is the semantic system? A critical review and meta-analysis of 120 functional neuroimaging studies. *Cerebral Cortex, 19*(12), 2767-2796.

Bishop, D. (2003). *Test for the Reception of Grammar (TROG)* (2nd ed.). London: Pearson.

Blom Johansson, M., Carlsson, M., Ostberg, P., & Sonnander, K. (2013). A multiple-case study of a family-oriented intervention practice in the early rehabilitation phase of persons with aphasia. *Aphasiology, 27*(2), 201-226.

Boller, F., & Green, E. (1972). Comprehension in severe aphasics. *Cortex, 8*(4), 382-394.

Bonini, M. V., & Radanovic, M. (2015). Cognitive deficits in post-stroke aphasia. *Arquivos de Neuro-Psiquiatria, 73*(10), 840-847.

Bonita, R., & Beaglehole, R. (1988). Recovery of motor function after stroke. *Stroke, 19*(12), 1497-1500.

Boyle, M. (2010). Semantic feature analysis treatment for aphasic word retrieval impairments: What's in a name? *Topics in Stroke Rehabilitation, 17*(6), 411-422.

Butt, P., & Bucks, P. (2004). *Butt Non-Verbal Reasoning Test*. Milton Keynes: Speechmark.

Cacciante, L., Kiper, P., Garzon, M., Baldan, F., Federico, S., Turolla, A., & Agostini, M. (2021, July-August). Telerehabilitation for people with aphasia: A systematic review and meta-analysis. *Journal of Communication Disorders, 92*, 106111.

Campbell, T. F., & McNeil, M. R. (1985). Effects of presentation rate and divided attention on auditory comprehension in children with an acquired language disorder. *Journal of Speech, Language, and Hearing Research, 28*(4), 513–520.

Caute, A., Roper, A., Dipper, L., & Pritchard, M. (2017). *City gesture checklist*. https://aphasia. talkbank.org/gesture/CGC.pdf

Centre for Evidence-based Medicine. (2009). *Levels of evidence.* www.cebm.net/2009/06/ oxford-centre-evidence-based-medicine-levels-evidence-march-2009/

Cherney, L. R., Patterson, J. P., & Raymer, A. M. (2011). Intensity of aphasia therapy: Evidence and efficacy. *Current Neurology and Neuroscience Reports, 11*(6), 560–569.

Cherney, L. R., & van Vuuren, S. (2012, August). Telerehabilitation, virtual therapists, and acquired neurologic speech and language disorders. *Seminars in Speech and Language, 33*(3), 243–257.

Chiou, H. S., & Kennedy, M. R. T. (2009). Switching in adults with aphasia. *Aphasiology, 23*(7–8), 1065–1075.

Choi, B. C. K., & Pak, A. W. P. (2006). Multidisciplinarity, interdisciplinarity and transdisciplinarity in health research, services, education and policy: Definitions, objectives, and evidence of effectiveness. *Clinical and Investigative Medicine, 29*(6), 351–364.

Clarke, M. T., Sargent, J., Cooper, R., Aberbach, G., McLaughlin, L., Panesar, G., . . . Swettenham, J. (2022). Development and testing of the eye-pointing classification scale for children with cerebral palsy. *Disability and Rehabilitation, 44*(8), 1451–1456.

Collins, M. (1986). *Diagnosis and treatment of global aphasia*. London: Taylor & Francis.

Conroy, P., Sage, K., & Lambon Ralph, M. A. (2009). Errorless and errorful therapy for verb and noun naming in aphasia. *Aphasiology, 23*(11), 1311–1337.

Cowan, N. (2010). The magical mystery four: How is working memory capacity limited, and why? *Current Directions in Psychological Science, 19*(1), 51–57.

Cuespeak Ltd (2022). *Cuespeak* (version 2.8.2) [Mobile app]. https://cuespeak.com/

Cumming, T. B., Marshall, R. S., & Lazar, R. M. (2013). Stroke, cognitive deficits, and rehabilitation: Still an incomplete picture. *International Journal of Stroke, 8*(1), 38–45.

Dabul, B. (2000). *Apraxia battery for adults-2*. Austin, TX: Pro-Ed.

Davis, G. A., & Wilcox, M. J. (1981). Incorporating parameters of natural conversation in aphasia treatment. In R. Chapey (Ed.), *Language intervention strategies in adult aphasia* (pp. 169–193). Baltimore: Williams & Wilkins.

Davis, G. A., & Wilcox, M. J. (1985). *Adult aphasia rehabilitation: Applied pragmatics*. Michigan: College-Hill Press.

De Brun, C. (2013). *Finding the evidence.* www.england.nhs.uk/tis/wp-content/uploads/sites/17/ 2014/09/tis-guide-finding-the-evidence-07nov.pdf

Denes, G., Perazzolo, C., Piani, A., & Piccione, F. (1996). Intensive versus regular speech therapy in global aphasia: A controlled study. *Aphasiology, 10*(4), 385–394.

De Renzi, E., Colombo, A., & Scarpa, M. (1991). The aphasic isolate: A clinical-CT scan study of a particularly severe subgroup of global aphasics. *Brain, 114*(4), 1719–1730.

De Renzi, E., & Vignolo, L. A. (1962). The token test: A sensitive test to detect receptive disturbances in aphasics. *Brain, 85*(4), 665–678.

Dick, F., Bates, E., Utman, J. A., Wulfeck, B., Dronkers, N., & Gernsbacher, M. A. (2001). Language deficits, localization, and grammar: Evidence for a distributive model of language breakdown in aphasic patients and neurologically intact individuals. *Psychological Review, 108*(4), 759–788.

Dignam, J., Copland, D., McKinnon, E., Burfein, P., O'Brien, K., Farrell, A., & Rodriguez, A. D. (2015). Intensive versus distributed aphasia therapy: A nonrandomized, parallel-group, dosage controlled study. *Stroke, 46*(8), 2206–2211.

Dorfler, E., & Kulnik, S. T. (2020). Despite communication and cognitive impairment person-centred goal-setting after a stroke: A qualitative study. *Disability and Rehabilitation, 42*(5), 3628–3637.

Dovern, A., Fink, G. R., & Weiss, P. H. (2012). Diagnosis and treatment of upper limb apraxia. *Journal of Neurology, 259,* 1269–1283.

Dressler, R. A. (2005). *LARK-2: Language activity resource kit* (2nd ed.). Austin: Pro Ed.

Dronkers, N. F., Plaisant, O., Iba-Zizen, M. T., & Cabanis, E. A. (2007). Paul Broca's historic cases: High resolution MR imaging of the brains of Leborgne and Lelong. *Brain, 130*(5), 1432–1441.

Duffy, J. R. (2005). *Motor speech disorders: Substrates, differential diagnosis and management* (2nd ed.). St Louis: Elsevier Mosby.

Duncan, J. (2010). The multiple-demand (MD) system of the primate brain: Mental programs for intelligent behaviour. *Trends in Cognitive Sciences, 14*(4), 172–179.

Edelman, G. (1987). Global aphasia: The case for treatment. *Aphasiology, 1*(1), 75–79.

El Hachioui, H., Visch-Brink, E. G., Lingsma, H. F., van de Sandt-Koenderman, M. W. M. E., Dippel, D. W. J., Koudstaal, P. J., & Middelkoop, H. A. M. (2014). Nonlinguistic cognitive impairment in poststroke aphasia: A prospective study. *Neurorehabilitation and Neural Repair, 28*(3), 273–281.

Ellis, A. W., & Young, A. W. (1996). *Human cognitive neuropsychology: A textbook with readings.* Hove: Psychology Press.

Erickson, R. J., Goldinger, S. D., & LaPointe, L. L. (1996). Auditory vigilance in aphasic individuals: Detecting non-linguistic stimuli with full or divided attention. *Brain and Cognition, 30*(2), 244–253.

Eriksen, B. A., & Eriksen, C. W. (1974). Effects of noise letters upon identification of a target letter in a nonsearch task. *Perception and Psychophysics, 16*, 143–149.

Ferro, J. M. (1992). The influence of infarct location on recovery from global aphasia. *Aphasiology, 6*(4), 415–430.

Fillingham, J. K., Hodgson, C., Sage, K., & Lambon Ralph, M. A. (2003). The application of errorless learning to aphasic disorders: A review of theory and practice. *Neuropsychological Rehabilitation, 13*(3), 337–363.

Frattali, C. M., Thompson, C. K., Holland, A., Wohl, C. B., & Ferketic, M. M. (1995). *American speech-language hearing association functional assessment of communication (ASHA-FACS).* Rockville: American Speech-Language Hearing Association.

Fridriksson, J., Nettles, C., Davis, M., Morrow, L., & Montgomery, A. (2006). Functional communication and executive function in aphasia. *Clinical Linguistics & Phonetics, 20*(6), 401–410.

Friedmann, N., & Gvion, A. (2003). Sentence comprehension and working memory limitation in aphasia: A dissociation between semantic-syntactic and phonological reactivation. *Brain and Language, 86*(1), 23–39.

Garrett, K. L., & Beukelman, D. R. (1998). Adults with severe aphasia. In D. R. Beukelman & P. Mirenda (Eds.), *Augmentative and alternative communication: Management of severe communication disorders in children and adults* (2nd ed., pp. 465–499). Baltimore: P.H. Brookes Publishing.

Garrett, K. L., & Lasker, J. P. (2005). *The multimodal communication screening task for persons with Aphasia; MCST-A.* https://cehs.unl.edu/documents/secd/aac/assessment/score.pdf

Geranmayeh, F., Brownsett, S. L. E., & Wise, R. J. S. (2014). Task-induced brain activity in aphasic stroke patients: What is driving recovery? *Brain, 137*(10), 2632–2648.

Glosser, G., & Goodglass, H. (1990). Disorders in executive control functions among aphasic and other brain-damaged patients. *Journal of Clinical and Experimental Neuropsychology, 12*(4), 485–501.

Goldberg, S., Haley, K. L., & Jacks, A. (2012). Script training and generalization for people with aphasia. *American Journal of Speech Language Pathology, 21*(3), 222–238.

Goll, J. C., Crutch, S. J., & Warren, J. D. (2010). Central auditory disorders: Toward a neuropsychology of auditory objects. *Current Opinion in Neurology, 23*(6), 617–627.

Goodglass, H. (1981). The syndromes of aphasia: Similarities and differences in neurolinguistic features. *Topics in Language Disorders, 1*(4), 1–14.

Goodglass, H., & Kaplan, E. (1972). *Boston diagnostic aphasia examination.* Philadelphia: Lea and Febiger.

Goodglass, H., Kaplan, E., & Barresi, B. (2001). *The Boston diagnostic aphasia examination: BDAE-3.* Philadelphia: Lippincott Williams & Wilkins.

Goodglass, H., Kaplan, E., & Brand, S. (1983). *The Boston diagnostic aphasia examination* (2nd ed.). Philadelphia: Lea and Febiger.

Grant, D. A., & Berg, E. (1948). A behavioral analysis of degree of reinforcement and ease of shifting to new responses in a Weigl-type card-sorting problem. *Journal of Experimental Psychology, 38*(4), 404–411.

Grant, D. A., & Berg, E. (1993). *Wisconsin card sorting test.* Florida: Psychological Assessment Resources.

Helm-Estabrooks, N. (1992). *ADP: Aphasia diagnostic profiles.* Austin: Pro-Ed.

Helm-Estabrooks, N. (2001). *Cognitive linguistic quick test: Examiner's manual.* Hove: Psychological Corp.

Helm-Estabrooks, N. (2002). Cognition and aphasia: A discussion and a study. *Journal of Communication Disorders, 35*, 171–186.

Helm-Estabrooks, N., & Albert, M. L. (2004). *Manual of aphasia and aphasia therapy* (2nd ed.). Austin: Pro-Ed.

Helm-Estabrooks, N., Albert, M. L., & Nicholas, M. (2014). *Manual of aphasia and aphasia therapy* (3rd ed.). Austin: Pro-Ed.

Helm-Estabrooks, N., Fitzpatrick, P. M., & Barresi, B. (1982). Visual action therapy for global aphasia. *Journal of Speech and Hearing Disorders, 47*(4), 385–389.

Helm-Estabrooks, N., & Holland, A. L. (1998). *Approaches to the treatment of aphasia*. San Diego: Singular Pub. Group.

Helm-Estabrooks, N., Ramsberger, G., Morgan, A. R., & Nicholas, M. (1989). *BASA: Boston assessment of severe aphasia*. Chicago: Riverside Publishing Company.

Herbert, R., Gregory, E., & Haw, C. (2019). Collaborative design of accessible information with people with aphasia. *Aphasiology, 33*(12), 1504-1530.

Hersch, D., Worrall, L., Howe, T., Sherratt, S., & Davidson, B. (2012). SMARTER goal setting in aphasia rehabilitation. *Aphasiology, 26*(2), 220-233.

Heuer, S., & Hallowell, B. (2007). An evaluation of multiple-choice test images for comprehension assessment in aphasia. *Aphasiology, 21*(9), 883-900.

Heuer, S., & Hallowell, B. (2009). Visual attention in a multiple-choice task: Influences of image characteristics with and without presentation of a verbal stimulus. *Aphasiology, 23*(3), 351-363.

Hier, D. B., Yoon, W. B., Mohr, J. P., Price, T. R., & Wolf, P. A. (1994). Gender and aphasia in the stroke data bank. *Brain and Language, 47*(1), 155-167.

Hilari, K., Byng, S., Lamping, D. L., & Smith, S. C. (2003). Stroke and aphasia quality of life scale-39 (SAQOL-39): Evaluation of acceptability, reliability, and validity. *Stroke, 34*(8), 1944-1950.

Hilari, K., & Dipper, L. (2020). *The scenario test (validated in the UK)*. Havant: J & R Press Ltd.

Hinckley, J., & Nash, C. (2007). Cognitive assessment and aphasia severity. *Brain and Language, 103*(1-2), 195-196.

Ho, K. M., Weiss, S. J., Garrett, K. L., & Lloyd, L. L. (2005). The effect of remnant and pictographic books on the communicative interaction of individuals with global aphasia. *Augmentative and Alternative Communication, 21*(3), 218-232.

Hoffman, T., Glasziou, P. P., Boutron, I., Milne, R., Moher, D., Altman, D., . . . Michie, S. (2014). Better reporting of interventions: Template for intervention description and replication (TIDieR) checklist and guide. *British Medical Jounral (BMJ), 348*, g1687.

Hogrefe, K., Ziegler, W., Weidinger, N., & Goldenberg, G. (2012). Non-verbal communication in severe aphasia: Influence of aphasia, apraxia or semantic processing? *Cortex, 48*, 952-962.

Holland, A., Frattali, C., & Fromm, D. (1999). *CADL-2: Communication activities of daily living*. Austin: Pro-Ed.

Holland, A. L. (1980). *CADL: Communicative abilities in daily living: A test of functional communication for aphasic adults*. Baltimore: University Park Press.

Holland, A. L., Fromm, D., & Wozniak, L. (2018). *CADL-3: Communication activities of daily living*. Austin: Pro-Ed.

Hoover, E. L., Caplan, D. N., Waters, G. S., & Carney, A. (2017). Communication and quality of life outcomes from an interprofessional intensive, comprehensive, aphasia program (ICAP). *Topics in Stroke Rehabilitation, 24*(2), 82-90.

Hope, T., Seghier, M., Leff, A., & Price, C. T. (2013). Predicting outcome and recovery after stroke with lesions extracted from MRI images. *Neuroimage: Clinical, 2*(1), 424-433.

Houghton, P., Towey, M. P., & Pettit, J. M. (1982). Measuring communication competence in global aphasia. *Clinical Aphasiology Conference Proceedings, 10*, 139-146.

Howard, D., & Patterson, K. (1992). *The pyramids and palm trees test: A test of semantic access from words and pictures*. Suffolk: Thames Valley Test Company.

Howe, T., Worrall, L., & Hickson, L. (2004). What is an aphasia friendly environment? *Aphasiology, 18*(11), 1015-1037.

Hubbard, H. I., Nelson, L. A., & Richardson, J. D. (2020). Can script training improve narrative and conversation in aphasia across etiology? *Seminars in Speech and Language, 41*(1), 99-124.

Humphreys, G. W., & Riddoch, M. J. (Eds.). (1987). *Visual object processing: A cognitive neuropsychological approach*. Hove: Lawrence Erlbaum Associates, Inc.

Ishigami, Y., & Klein, R. M. (2011). Repeated measurement of the components of attention of older adults using the two versions of the Attention Network Test: Stability, isolability, robustness, and reliability. *Frontiers in Aging Neuroscience, 3*, 17.

Kagan, A. (1999). *Supported conversation for adults with aphasia*. [Doctoral thesis, University of Toronto]. https://tspace.library.utoronto.ca/bitstream/1807/12973/1/NQ45755.pdf

Kagan, A., Simmons-Mackie, N., Rowland, A., Huijbregts, M., Shumway, E., McEwen, S., . . . Sharp, S. (2008). Counting what counts: A framework for capturing real-life outcomes of aphasia intervention. *Aphasiology, 22*(3), 258-280.

Kalbe, E., Reinhold, N., Brand, M., Markowitsch, H. J., & Kessler, J. (2005). A new test battery to assess aphasic disturbances and associated cognitive dysfunctions: German normative data on the Aphasia Check List. *Journal of Clinical and Experimental Neuropsychology, 27*(7), 779-794.

Kaschak, M. P., Madden, C. J., Therriault, D. J., Yaxley, R. H., Aveyard, M., Blanchard, A. A., & Zwaan, R. A. (2005). Perception of motion affects language processing. *Cognition, 94*(3), 79-89.

Kaye, R. C., & Cherney, L. R. (2016). Script templates: A practical approach to script training in aphasia. *Topics in Language Disorders, 36*(2), 136-153.

Keil, K., & Kaszniak, A. W. (2002). Examining executive function in individuals with brain injury: A review. *Aphasiology, 16*(3), 305-335.

Kertesz, A. (2006). *Western aphasia battery revised.* San Antonio: Pearson.

Kertesz, A., & McCabe, P. (1975). Intelligence and aphasia: Performance of aphasics on Raven's Coloured Progressive Matrices (RCPM). *Brain and Language, 2,* 387-395.

Keyserling, A. G., Naujokat, C., Niemann, W., Huber, W., & Thron, A. (1997). Global aphasia - with and without hemiparesis: A linguistic and CT scan study. *European Neurology, 38,* 259-267.

Kluding, P. M., Tseng, B. Y., & Billinger, S. A. (2011). Exercise and executive function in individuals with chronic stroke. *Journal of Neurologic Physical Therapy, 35*(1), 11-17.

Kohs, S. C. (1920). The block-design tests. *Journal of Experimental Psychology, 3*(5), 357-376.

Kongs, S. K., Thompson, L. L., Iverson, G. L., & Heaton, R. K. (2000). *Wisconsin card sorting test-64 card version.* Florida: Par Inc.

Koul, R., Corwin, M., & Hayes, S. (2004). Production of graphic symbol sentences by individuals with aphasia: Efficacy of a computer-based augmentative and alternative communication intervention. *Brain and Language, 92,* 58-77.

Lasker, J. P., & Garrett, K. L. (2006). Using the Multimodal Communication Screening Test for Persons with Aphasia (MCST-A) to guide the selection of alternative communication strategies for people with aphasia. *Aphasiology, 20*(2-4), 217-232.

Law, M., Baptiste, S., Carswell, A., McColl, M. A., Polatajko, H. J., & Pollock, N. (2019). *Canadian occupational performance measure* (5th ed.). Altona: COPM Inc.

Lawson, R., & Fawcus, M. (1999). Increasing effective communication using a total communication approach. In S. Byng, K. Swinburn, & C. Pound (Eds.), *The aphasia therapy file: Volume 1.* Hove: Psychology Press.

Leff, A. P., Nightingale, S., Gooding, B., Rutter, J,. Craven, N., Peart, M., . . . Crinion, J. T. (2021). Clinical effectiveness of the Queen Square intensive comprehensive aphasia service for patients with poststroke aphasia. *Stroke, 52*(10), 594-598.

Leff, A. P., Schofield, T. M., Crinion, J. T., Seghier, M. L., Grogan, A., Green, D. W., & Price, C. J. (2009). The left superior temporal gyrus is a shared substrate for auditory short-term memory and speech comprehension: Evidence from 210 patients with stroke. *Brain, 132*(12), 3401-3410.

Lock, S., Wilkinson, R., Bryan, K., Maxim, J., Edmundson, A., Bruce, C., & Moir, D. (2001). Supporting Partners of People with Aphasia in Relationships and Conversation (SPPARC). *International Journal of Language and Communication Disorders, 36,* S25-30.

Long, A., Hesketh, A., & Bowen, A. (2009). Communication outcome after stroke: A new measure of the carer's perspective. *Clinical Rehabilitation, 23,* 846-856.

Lubinski, R. (1981). Environmental language intervention. In R. Chapey (Ed.), *Language intervention strategies in adult aphasia* (pp. 223-245). Baltimore: Williams & Wilkins.

Luzzatti, C., Willmes, K., & De Bleser, R. (1991). *Aachener aphasie test versione Italiana.* Florence: Organizzazioni Speciali.

Magee, W. L. (2019). Why include music therapy in a neurorehabilitation team? *Advances in Clinical Neuroscience and Rehabilitation.* https://doi.org/10.47795/STUI1319

Maguire, A., Nicholas, M., & Zipse, L. (2012). *Cognitive flexibility: A new assessment.* Poster presented at the ASHA Convention, Atlanta, Georgia.

Malia, K., & Brannagan, A. (2014). *Cognitive rehabilitation workshop for professionals.* Surrey: Brain Tree Training.

Marinelli, C. V., Spaccavento, S., Craca, A., Marangolo, P., & Angelelli, P. (2017). Different cognitive profiles of patients with severe aphasia. *Behavioural Neurology,* 1-15.

Marshall, R. (1987a). Reapportioning time for aphasia rehabilitation: A point of view: Reply to Wertz, Edelman and Parsons. *Aphasiology, 1,* 91-95.

Marshall, R. (1987b). Reapportioning time for aphasia rehabilitation: A point of view. *Aphasiology, 1,* 59-73.

Mark, V. W., Thomas, B. E., & Derndt, R. S. (1992). Factors associated with improvement in global aphasia. *Aphasiology, 6*(2), 121-134.

Mattheiss, S. R., Levinson, H., & Graves, W. W. (2018). Duality of function: Activation for meaningless nonwords and semantic codes in the same brain areas. *Cerebral Cortex, 28*(7), 2516-2524.

McCall, D., Shelton, J. R., Weinrich, M., & Cox, D. (2000). The utility of computerized visual communication for improving natural language in chronic global aphasia: Implications for approaches to treatment in global aphasia. *Aphasiology, 14*(8), 795–826.

Mental Capacity Act. (2005). www.legislation.gov.uk/ukpga/2005/9/pdfs/ukpga_20050009_en.pdf

Meteyard, L., Bahrami, B., & Vigliocco, G. (2007). Motion detection and motion verbs: Language affects low-level visual perception. *Psychological Science, 18*(11), 1007–1013.

Milan University Neuropsychology Center. (1974). *Milan language examination.* Florence: Organizzazioni Speciali.

Mineroff, Z., Blank, I. A., Mahowald, K., & Fedorenko, E. (2018). A robust dissociation among the language, multiple demand, and default mode networks: Evidence from inter-region correlations in effect size. *Neuropsychologia, 119*, 501–511.

Miyake, A., & Friedman, N. P. (2012). The nature and organisation of individual differences in executive functions: Four general conclusions. *Current Directions in Psychological Science, 21*(1), 8–14.

Monnelly, K., Marshall, J., & Cruice, M. (2021). Intensive comprehensive aphasia programmes: A systematic scoping review and analysis using the TIDieR checklist for reporting interventions. *Disability and Rehabilitation*, ahead-of-print, 1–26. doi:10.1080/09638288.2021.1964626

Morrow-Odom, K. L., & Swann, A. B. (2013). Effectiveness of melodic intonation therapy in a case of aphasia following right hemisphere stroke. *Aphasiology, 27*(11), 1322–1338.

Munro, P., & Siyambalapitiya, S. (2016). Improved word comprehension in global aphasia using a modified semantic feature analysis treatment. *Clinical Linguistics & Phonetics, 31*(2), 119–136.

Murphy, J. (1998a). Helping people with severe communication difficulties to express their views: A low-tech tool. *Communication Matters, 12*(2), 9–11.

Murphy, J. (1998b). Talking mats: Speech and language research in practice. *Speech and Language Therapy in Practice, Autumn 1998*, 11–14.

Murphy, J., & Boa, S. (2012). Using the WHO-ICF with talking mats as a goal setting tool. *Augmentative and Alternative Communication, 28*(1), 52–60.

Murray, L. (2017). Focusing attention on executive functioning in aphasia. *Aphasiology, 31*(7), 721–724.

Murray, L., Holland, A., & Beeson, P. (1997). Accuracy monitoring and task demand evaluation in aphasia. *Aphasiology, 11*(4–5), 410–414.

Murray, L., Salis, C., Martin, N., & Dralle, J. (2018). The use of standardised short-term and working memory tests in aphasia research: A systematic review. *Neuropsychological Rehabilitation, 28*(3), 309–351.

Nagaratnam, N., & McNeil, C. (1999). Dementia in the severely aphasic: Global aphasia without hemiparesis: A stroke subtype simulating dementia. *American Journal of Alzheimer's Disease, 14*(2), 74–78.

Nicholas, M., & Connor, L. T. (2017). People with aphasia using AAC: Are executive functions important? *Aphasiology, 31*(7), 819–836.

Olsson, C., Arvidsson, P., & Blom Johansson, M. (2019). Relations between executive function, language, and functional communication in severe aphasia. *Aphasiology, 33*(7), 821–845.

Porch, B. E. (1967). *Porch index of communicative ability.* California: Consulting Psychologists Press.

Purdy, M. (2002). Executive function ability in persons with aphasia. *Aphasiology, 16*(4–6), 549–557.

Purdy, M., & Van Dyke, J. A. (2011). Multimodal communication training in aphasia: A pilot study. *Journal of Medical Speech-Language Pathology, 19*(2), 43–53.

Purdy, M., & Wallace, S. E. (2016). Intensive multimodal communication treatment for people with chronic aphasia. *Aphasiology, 30*(10), 1071–1093.

Raven, J. C. (1956). *Coloured progressive matrices.* Oxford: Oxford Psychologist Press.

Raven, J. C., Court, J. H., & Raven, J. (1990). *Raven's coloured progressive matrices.* Oxford: Oxford Psychology Press.

Rende, B. (2000). Cognitive flexibility: Theory, assessment, and treatment. *Seminars in Speech and Language, 21*(2), 121–132.

Robin, D., & Rizzo, M. (1989). The effect of focal cerebral lesions on intramodal and cross-modal orienting of attention. *Clinical Aphasiology, 18*, 61–74.

Rönnberg, J., Larsson, C., Fogelsjöö, A., Nilsson, L. G., Lindberg, M., & Ängquist, K. A. (1996). Memory dysfunction in mild aphasics. *Scandinavian Journal of Psychology, 37*(1), 46–61.

Rose, M. L., Cherney, L. R., & Worrall, L. E. (2013). Intensive comprehensive aphasia programs: An international survey of practice. *Topics in Stroke Rehabilitation, 20*(5), 379–387.

Royal College of Physicians (RCP) Intercollegiate Stroke Working Party. (2016). *National clinical guideline for stroke* (5th ed.). Royal College of Physicians. https://www.strokeaudit.org/SupportFiles/Documents/Guidelines/2016-National-Clinical-Guideline-for-Stroke-5t-(1).aspx, (strokeaudit.org).

Sacchett, C., Byng, S., Marshall, J., & Pound, C. (1999). Drawing together: Evaluation of a therapy programme for severe aphasia. *International Journal of Language and Communication Disorders, 34*(3), 265-268.

Saldert, C., Backman, E., & Hartelius, L. (2013). Conversation partner training with spouses of persons with aphasia: A pilot study using a protocol to trace relevant characteristics. *Aphasiology, 27*(3), 271-292.

Samples, J. M., & Lane, V. W. (1980). Language gains in global aphasia over a three year period: A case study. *Journal of Communication Disorders, 13*, 49-57.

Sarno, M. T. (1969). *The functional communication profile.* New York: Institute of Rehabilitation Medicine.

Sarno, M. T., & Levita, E. (1981). Some observations on the nature of recovery in global aphasia after stroke. *Brain and Language, 13*(1), 1-12.

Schuell, H., Jenkins, J. J., & Jimenez-Pabon, E. (1964). *Aphasia in adults.* New York: Harper and Row.

Shallice, T. (1982). Specific impairments of planning. *Philosophical Transactions of the Royal Society B: Biological Sciences, 298*(1089), 199-209.

Simic, T., Rochon, E., Greco, E., & Martino, R. (2019). Baseline executive control ability and its relationship to language therapy improvements in post-stroke aphasia: A systematic review. *Neuropsychological Rehabilitation, 29*(3), 395-439.

Simon, H. A. (1975). The functional equivalence of problem-solving skills. *Cognitive Psychology, 7*(2), 268-288.

Simons, J. S., & Lambon Ralph, M. A. (1999). The auditory agnosias. *Neurocase, 5*(5), 379-406.

Slevc, L. R., & Shell, A. R. (2015). Auditory agnosia. In J. Katz, M. Chasin, K. M. English, L. J. Hood, & K. L. Tillery (Eds.), *Handbook of clinical audiology* (7th ed., pp. 573-587). Philadelphia: Wolters Kluwer Health.

Smania, N., Gandolfi, M., Aglioti, S. M., Girardi, P., Fiaschi, A., & Girardi, F. (2010). How long is the recovery of global aphasia? Twenty-five years of follow-up in a patient with left hemisphere stroke. *Neurorehabilitation and Neural Repair, 24*(9), 871-875.

Snaphaan, L., & de Leeuw, F. E. (2007). Poststroke memory function in nondemented patients: A systematic review on frequency and neuroimaging correlates. *Stroke, 38*(1), 198-203.

Sohlberg, M. M., & Mateer, C. A. (1987). Effectiveness of an attention-training program. *Journal of Clinical and Experimental Neuropsychology, 9*(2), 117-130.

Speechmark. (2004a). *Indoor sounds: Colorcards.* Milton Keynes: Speechmark Publishing Ltd.

Speechmark. (2004b). *Outdoor sounds: Colorcards.* Milton Keynes: Speechmark Publishing Ltd.

Speechmark. (2012). *Everyday objects: Colorcards.* Milton Keynes: Speechmark Publishing Ltd.

Stans, S. E. A., Dalemans, R. J. P., de Witte, L. P., Smeets, H. W. H., & Beurskens, A. J. (2017). The role of the physical environment in conversations between people who are communication vulnerable and health-care professionals: A scoping review. *Disability and Rehabilitation, 39*(25), 2594-2605.

Swinburn, K., Byng, S., & Firenza, C. (2006). *The communication disability profile.* London: Connect Press.

Swinburn, K., Porter, G., & Howard, D. (2004). *CAT: Comprehensive aphasia test.* Hove: Psychology Press.

Tactus Therapy Solutions Ltd. (2022a). *Language therapy* (version 2.07) [Mobile app]. https://tactustherapy.com/app/language

Tactus Therapy Solutions Ltd. (2022b). *Category therapy* (version 2.05) [Mobile app]. https://tactustherapy.com/app/category

Tactus Therapy Solutions Ltd. (2022c). *Advanced naming therapy* (version 2.07) [Mobile app]. https://tactustherapy.com/app/advanced-naming/

Thaut, C. P. (2016). Symbolic Communication Training through Music (SYCOM). In M. H. Thaut & V. Hoemberg (Eds.), *Handbook of neurologic music therapy* (pp. 216-220). Oxford: Oxford University Press.

Thaut, M. H. (2005). *Neurologic music therapy techniques and definitions.* https://nmtacademy.files.wordpress.com/2015/07/nmt-definitions.pdf

Tseng, C. H., McNeil, M. M., & Milenkovic, P. (1993). An investigation of attention allocation deficits in aphasia. *Brain and Language, 45*(2), 276-296.

University College London (UCL). (2020). *Eye-pointing classification scale.* www.ucl.ac.uk/gaze/sites/gaze/files/eye-pointing_classification_scale_2020_final.pdf

Van Mourik, M., Verschaeve, M., Boon, P., Paquier, P., & van Harskamp, F. (1992). Cognition in global aphasia: Indicators for therapy. *Aphasiology, 6*(5), 491-499.

Villard, S., & Kiran, S. (2015). Between-session intra-individual variability in sustained, selective, and integrational non-linguistic attention in aphasia. *Neuropsychologia, 66*, 204-212.

Villard, S., & Kiran, S. (2017). To what extent does attention underlie language in aphasia? *Aphasiology, 31*(10), 1226-1245.

Villard, S., & Kiran, S. (2018). Between-session and within-session intra-individual variability in attention in aphasia. *Neuropsychologia, 109,* 95-106.

Wallace, S. E., Purdy, M., & Skidmore, E. (2014). A multimodal communication program for aphasia during inpatient rehabilitation: A case study. *NeuroRehabilitation, 35*(3), 615-625.

Wapner, W., & Gardner, H. (1979). A note on patterns of comprehension and recovery in global aphasia. *Journal of Speech Language and Hearing Research, 22*(4), 765.

Ward-Lonergan, J. M., & Nicholas, M. (1995). Drawing to communicate: A case report of an adult with global aphasia. *European Journal of Disorders of Communication, 30*(4), 475-491.

Warren, M. (1993). A hierarchical model for evaluation and treatment of visual perceptual dysfunction in adult acquired brain injury, Part 1. *American Journal of Occupational Therapy, 47*(1), 42-54.

Wechsler, D. (1955). *Wechsler adult intelligence scale.* New York: The Psychological Corporation.

Weintraub, S., Dikmen, S. S., Heaton, R. K., Tulsky, D. S., Zelazo, P. D., Bauer, P. J., . . . Gershon, R. C. (2013). Cognition assessment using the NIH toolbox. *Neurology, 12;*80(11 Suppl 3), S54-64.

Whurr, R. (2011). *Aphasia screening test: A multi-dimensional assessment procedure for adults with acquired aphasia* (3rd ed.). Milton Keynes: Speechmark Publishing.

Woolf, C., Caute, A., Haigh, Z., Galliers, J., Wilson, S., Kessie, A., Hirani, S., Hegarty, B., & Marshall, J. (2016). A comparison of remote therapy, face to face therapy and an attention control intervention for people with aphasia: A quasi-randomised controlled feasibility study. *Clinical Rehabilitation, 30*(4), 359-373.

World Health Organisation. (2001). *International classification of functioning, disability, and health: ICF.* Geneva: World Health Organization.

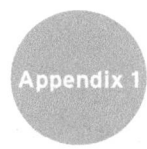

EXAMPLE COMMUNICATION HISTORY FORM

It is helpful to know as much as possible about clients, their family, their work, and their interests, as this helps tailor assessment and therapy to their individual communication needs. Please answer the following questions with as much detail as you feel comfortable with on behalf of your relative.

Client's name	
What do they prefer to be called?	
What is their date of birth?	
What is their first language?	
What, other languages do they speak, if any?	
Where and with whom do they live or did they live?	
Where were they born? Where have they lived in the past?	
Do they wear glasses?	
Do they have any hearing issues?	

	Name(s)	Where They Live
Spouse/partner		
Children/stepchildren		

Grandchildren/great-grandchildren		
Siblings		
Other close relatives		
Friends		

Please give the name(s) and details of any pet(s) owned now or in the past.

Were they working before becoming ill? If so, in what role and where?

If not, were they retired or unemployed? What roles have they held in the past?

What are their religious beliefs, if any? Do they worship regularly?

What do or did they enjoy as a hobby?

What sports did they play or watch? What is their favourite team, if any?

What type of music do they like? Who is their favourite band or singer?

What type of music do they dislike?

What type of television programmes or films do they enjoy?

What particular genres of television show or film do they dislike?

What are their favourite foods and drinks?

What foods and drinks do they dislike?

If you are able, please give a summary of a typical day for your relative. (e.g. where they might go, who they might speak to, what they might do and at what times of day)

What particular places do they or did they like to visit? What are or were their regular holiday destinations?

How would you describe their personality?

What topics do they like to talk about?

What topics are best avoided? (e.g. if they may trigger strong emotions or upset your relative)

Are or were they computer literate? Did they use iPads/tablets/apps, etc.?

_____

Is there anything else you would like us to know about your relative?

_____

THANK YOU FOR COMPLETING THIS QUESTIONNAIRE

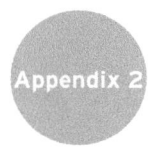

EXAMPLE OF AN AUTOMATIC SPEECH TASK

As discussed in Chapter 3, it is important that a client's cultural and linguistic background is taken into account when selecting the phrases to use in such a task as well as when analysing and scoring the client's response. Check with relatives which contexts are likely to be very familiar to their loved one or whether they can think of other very familiar sayings the client may have used or heard regularly.

The aim is for the SaLT to provide the phrase on the left and the client to complete this with an appropriate target. Suggested targets are provided but appropriate alternatives the client may be more familiar with should be accepted.

If a client has retained some reading abilities, it can be useful to compare performance when only the verbal cue is provided with performance when the verbal and written cues are presented together.

Therapist Cue	Client Target
A cup of	tea
Talk on the	phone
Son and	daughter
Pen and	paper
Watch the	telly
Table and	chair
Sleep in a	bed
Open the	window
A loaf of	bread
....	....

EXAMPLE OF A VISUAL SCALE

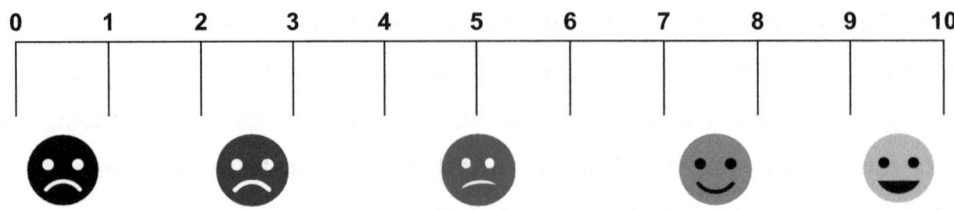

Figure A3.1 An example of a visual mood chart with severity depicted by numerical levels, facial expression, and shading of the emoji

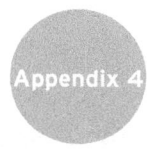

STRATEGIES FOR COMMUNICATING WITH PWGA

- Limit background noise by ensuring doors and windows are closed and televisions or radios are switched off.
- Remove any visual distractions from the person's immediate eye line.
- Maximise lighting to ensure the person can clearly see the speaker's face for interpreting facial expressions.
- Face the person and maintain eye contact.
- Use short phrases of three or four words rather than full sentences.
- Use short words and basic vocabulary.
- Emphasise the main words in sentences. For example, "**Anita** has gone **shopping**."
- Pause between sentences.
- Try to communicate about concrete topics occurring in real time.
- Point at objects, people, or pictures to aid the person's understanding of who or what is being referred to.
- If a more complex topic is being discussed, provide a relevant image or drawing to aid the person's comprehension.
- Be explicit when a topic is changing by removing the image or drawing, saying "finished," and using a relevant gesture to illustrate this.
- Be explicit when asking a question that you would like the person to respond to. For example, say "**Question** for **you**" whilst simultaneously pointing to them before or after asking a short question with simplified language.
- Use a normal tone of voice.
- Avoid speaking louder or significantly more slowly.
- Ask questions that require only a "yes" or "no" answer.
- Encourage the person to use a Yes/No chart if verbal responses are inconsistent.
- Check the person's responses by repeating a yes/no question at least twice, as many PwGA confuse these concepts.
- Give examples or forced choice. For example, "Do you want tea or coffee?" or "Is it X or Y?"
- Encourage the person to use picture communication charts to respond.
- Give the person extra time to respond.
- Use mime/gesture (along with simple language) to aid the person's comprehension.

- Try writing key words but be aware reading can be just as difficult for PwGA as understanding spoken words.
- Avoid asking the person to repeat words unnecessarily.
- Avoid asking "test questions" that you already know the answer to, which can be patronising.
- If communicating an idea is getting frustrating, leave it and come back to the issue later.

Index